BEST BODY™

cookbook
& menu plan

Sohailla Digsby, RDN, LD & Kim Beavers, MS, RDN, LD, CDE

Sid – To your delicious health!
Kim B. ☺

YOU'RE
AWAY
FROM YOUR
BEST BODY

52 DAYS

Published by Western Wall Press

Best Body™ Countdown and the 52 Days™ are trademarks of Sohailla Digsby.

ISBN: 978-0-692-60301-7
Copyright © Sohailla Digsby and Kim Beavers
Recipe Photography by Kim Beavers
Book Cover & Text Design by Summer R. Morris

Printed in the United States of America
2016

5 vegetable and fruit servings or more daily

4 cook-at-home meals weekly+

3 "Strategic Splurges" per week

2 meals from 1 (double recipes)

1 hour of pre-prep and planning time weekly

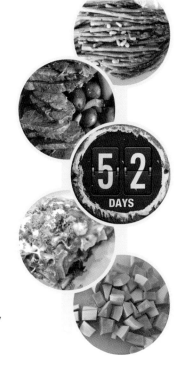

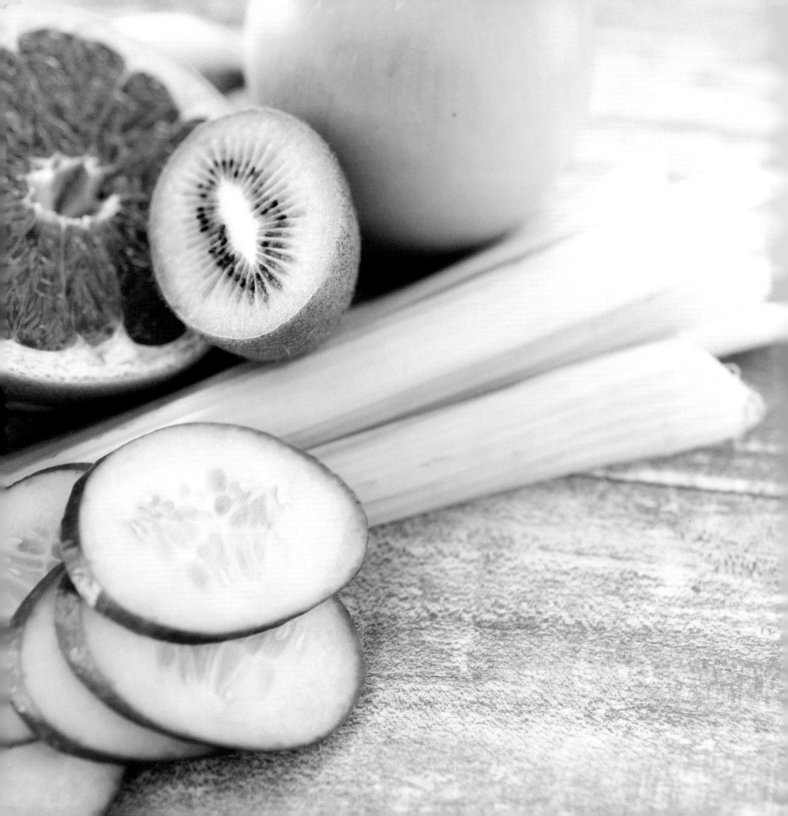

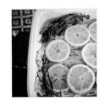 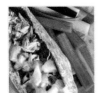 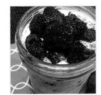 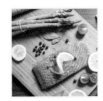

contents

"Abs are made

in the kitchen"

—UNKNOWN

Your Best Body

We are not just about giving you delicious recipes, menus and cooking tips, though *we will!* Our goal is to equip you with meals tasting so good that you feel confident you'll be able to reach and maintain Your Best Body. If your current pursuit is that of delicious, wholesome recipes, but you don't see yourself making lifestyle changes to reach Your Best Body anytime soon, we appreciate you being realistic. As dietitians, we know your personal readiness is key. We hope to inspire and motivate you to choose what is Best for *your* Body as you turn these pages and serve our favorite recipes in your home. We will be setting you up for success whether your goal is to lose weight over the next 52 days, to simplify your evenings with set menu plans, or to be satisfied with the flavor that well-prepared, healthful food offers.

If you are looking for an extreme diet fix, a detox that has you dragging for a number of days, or a meal plan that is only realistic to maintain for a month, this is not it. However, if you are looking for fabulous recipes for any time and any physique, a menu plan that does the nutrition calculations for you, increased confidence in the kitchen, and flavorful foods that will help you to reach Your Best Body, then you have the perfect success tool in hand! This book is the fulfillment of countless requests for daily recipes and menu-planning guidance to go along with the daily challenges of the ***Countdown to Your Best Body Success Journal*** that I (Sohailla) wrote not long ago.

Kim and I believe in balance and moderation as well as the joy of cooking and eating, provided the latter is not at the expense of one's health. Being Your Best is not *just* about a bikini-ready body (though that certainly is a realistic ambition for the next 52 days). Being Your Best is about feeling comfortable in your own skin *and* last year's wardrobe; it's about being in control when it comes to food, and being fueled well enough to live energetically (not to mention to ward off headaches, fatigue, and the many medical complications related to food choices).

With more than 30 years of experience as dietitians between us, we are not fazed by fads or inspired by extremes. Our intention is for those who enjoy our recipes to reach and maintain their Best Bodies for a lifetime. That said, we are fine with serving meat at mealtime, as long as it doesn't take up half your plate; we are not scared of carbs at meals (gasp!), as long as they don't load half your plate, and we are not worried about you having a pat of butter, as long it doesn't end up coating half your plate. You see where I am going with this: over time, what you put on half of your plate affects the whole of your life. Both balance and moderation are critical to a consistently healthy lifestyle.

We are going to be focusing on what matters *most* and keeps you consistently at Your Best Body (not just for your class reunion weekend). I have had clients ask me if bananas are making them fat, meanwhile they eat out every day for lunch...bananas are not likely the issue. They ask me about what to sprinkle in their water to make it yummy, meanwhile they hardly take in enough water to rehydrate because they don't bother to perspire (aka move) much...their water flavor is not likely their problem. They ask me for healthy menus like the ones we provide here, but oftentimes their meals are not the problem either. Typically it's the weekend "well-deserved splurges" or what they've allowed to jump in the grocery cart that accosts them between meals when they've gotten too hungry, or late-night treats when the long hours of the day have worn down their will. While we are doing our part to give you the recipes and tools you need to be Your Best, it is equally important that you make choices outside of your mealtimes that support your Best-Body efforts in the kitchen.

> For many, reaching Your Best Body destination requires weight loss. Weight lost during this Countdown will not be water weight or muscle weight—just the fluffy, jiggly, over-your-waistband kind of stuff that you want gone. It would be wrong of me to encourage weight loss strategies that have you reaching Your Best Body goal weight by way of dehydration, diarrhea, and muscle atrophy. I know that you want the numbers to drop fast, but I don't want my 52-day Countdown *winners* to be dehydrated, mushy-muscle "losers".

Excerpt from the *Countdown to Your Best Body Success Journal,* page 9

So, trust the process, and when you need encouragement to stay strong, take a moment to read the clips throughout this book, as well as the Success Stories of the others who have gone before you (bestbodyin52.com). Keep in mind that the discoveries these "Best Body Superstars" made about what needed to change in order to be successful required the use of the Success Journal, and often more than one 52-day round.

Fitness Pro meets Foodie

We had a blast writing this book together (honestly, no fights)! We combine two totally different RDN backgrounds to bring a balanced approach to you. I (Sohailla) work with active clients seeking to manage their weight, and train facilitators around the country to utilize the Best Body Countdown program I created with groups in their gyms and worksites. Cooking for my active family is a joy, but not part of my work directly. As a fitness pro, I love being in the gym as much as the kitchen. I thought I was a bit of a foodie until I met Kim and realized how many different textures of salt a true foodie has on hand, for example.

Kim works elbow-deep in food, developing and tweaking recipes and then cleans up the kitchen to go on camera for her weekly televised culinary nutrition segment, *Eating Well with Kim*. As a recipe developer, she can often be found in the kitchen or the grocery store. Fitness for her is a joy, but is not part of her work directly. As you might imagine, we learned a lot from each other while putting together this cookbook and look forward to hearing about what you learn over these next 52 days as well.

Share something you learn on the Best Body in 52 Facebook page!

For Kim, a jog is nice, but for me, a jog with 30-second sprint intervals mixed in is far more invigorating. For me, a roast with fresh garlic and cracked pepper is nice, but for Kim, that same roast marinated, seared, and seasoned with hearty herbs is far more enjoyable. We had your vitality *and* your taste buds in mind while putting together these recipes and guidelines to help you to be Your Best, not to mention your budget and your busy schedule. Kim and I are real-life multitasking moms who love good food and the vivacity it provides, so we will only ask of you what we are willing and able to do ourselves.

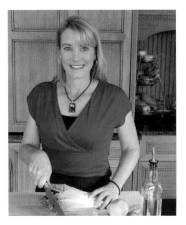

Kim in her home kitchen

The Best Body Countdown recipes are strategically ordered to be paired with the challenges laid out in my **Countdown to Your Best Body Success Journal** over 52 days. As your biggest fans along Your Best Body journey, Kim and I have thought through every detail on your behalf, providing recipes, menus and guidance so you can check off the Countdown challenges in your Success Journal with confidence. However, if you are not participating in the 52-day Countdown at this time, you can certainly still learn from the many practical health-promoting tips we offer.

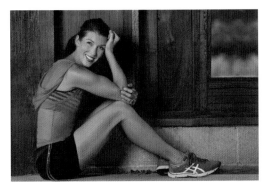

Sohailla on the bridge she jogs over regularly

RECIPE AND MENU PLAN OVERVIEW

Our recipes will meet your nutrition needs without discounting the importance of flavor or convenience. They are fairly simple and take an average of 30 minutes to prepare. Some evenings, you may just choose one of the recipes off the menu, and for others, you may want

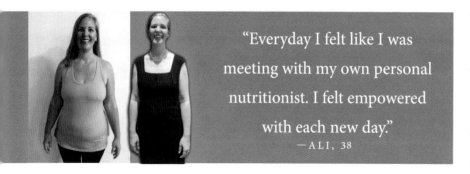

"Everyday I felt like I was meeting with my own personal nutritionist. I felt empowered with each new day."
—ALI, 38

to invite company for a phenomenal spread. We encourage you to use this cookbook and menu plan to make the next 52 days Your Best!

The next several pages outline everything you'll need to get both you and your kitchen set up for success to start the Best Body Countdown, a 52-day lifestyle-change journey with the result being you at Your Best Body! By the end of the Countdown, you'll have a pantry and medical profile that look as different from 52 days ago as you do in your jeans. So, if your goal is to make a change in you, and not just your recipe box, you'll want to keep a copy of the **Success Journal** on hand. If not, the recipes are just as delicious!

In this cookbook and menu plan, you will get a weekly dinner menu for the first six weeks of the Countdown. Over the final two weeks, you'll wrap up by developing a two-week menu of your favorite Best Body recipes to continue until the completion of the Countdown, setting yourself up for Best-Body success that goes far beyond 52 days.

To help you keep the essentials in mind that will direct you on the path to Your Best Body, you'll want to commit the following **Cookbook Countdown 5-4-3-2-1** to memory.

Though we have provided daily dinner recipes each week for you, we don't expect you to cook every night of the week. However, we do suggest that you prepare at least four of your evening meals at home per week, building them around produce as the priority, and doubling recipes, so you'll have plenty for healthy "Lunch Leftovers" and dinners throughout the week.

We have your meals covered, but we would be remiss if we didn't address what

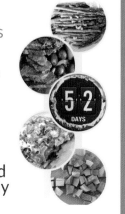

5 vegetable and fruit servings or more daily

4 cook-at-home meals weekly+

3 "Strategic Splurges" per week

2 meals from 1 (double recipes)

1 hour of pre-prep and planning time weekly

"happens" between meals and on special occasions. Splurges are certainly part of a full life, but if they are not strategic, mindful splurges, they will throw you off course, deterring you from your Best-Body goals. At the start of each week, we suggest you determine three weekly "Strategic Splurges" that

Take a moment to test yourself: how close are you to stating the **Cookbook Countdown 5-4-3-2-1** from memory?

won't sabotage your goals. Lastly, we will teach you how to make the most of one hour of pre-prep and planning time weekly so that you don't find the pizza delivery guy at your door on the days that follow. Each of these five concepts will be reiterated over the next 52 days until they are second nature to you.

So, are you ready to make your kitchen the central hub of Your Best-Body success? You'll need to understand the upcoming terms and utilize the suggested tools and tips that follow in order to get the most out of this book… resist the temptation to skip straight to the recipes: you'll be enjoying them bite by delicious bite soon enough!

> " Motivation is a fire from within."
> —STEPHEN COVEY

Terms, Tools and Tips

Terms

My definition of *clean eating* for the Best Body Countdown:

› You don't have to clean the grease-based lip gloss off your lips between bites (think lo mein).

› You do have to clean out your fridge if you go out of town because most of the food is perishable.

› You don't have to clean your pizza, that is, you don't have to use your napkin to sop up the fat that puddles on the top (ewww).

› No need to clean salt granules off your table or worry about how much sodium is in everything because so few of your foods are packaged, canned, or cured that the small amount of sodium you are getting from the real food you are eating is no big deal. (Hint: if it has a flavoring packet or is pre-seasoned, it is likely very high in sodium).

› It won't be as tough to clean your frying pan because the lean meats you are using won't leave a saturated mess in the pan.

› Your body "takes out the trash" every day because your daily fiber-filled foods, your 64+ ounces of real water, and your exercise are cleaning things out (need I be more specific?).

› You don't have to take medications to clean the buildup out of your arteries because your food sources containing soluble fiber prevent your digestive system from absorbing cholesterol.

menu key:

Lunch Leftovers   Pricey Meal   Quicker-Fix   Slow-Cooker   Club Favorite   Easy Meal

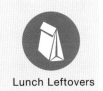

Lunch Leftovers

This icon will be shown on the dinner menus to indicate which recipes we suggest as "Lunch Leftovers." We encourage you to eat food from home for lunch as often as possible. We don't give a specific menu lineup for lunch because, in our experience as registered dietitians, we've learned that most people don't cook from recipes at lunchtime. Most either serve up leftovers at home, grab a sandwich on the go, or eat lunch out. You will find many fabulous lunch options in this book, just not in the form of a lunch menu.

Slow-Cooker

This icon will be shown whenever a slow cooker is used to prepare a meal—at least once a week to minimize your kitchen time. Because these meals are often started in the morning, this icon will give you forward notice, so you can make the best use of your Slow-Cooker as well as your time.

Easy Meal

Most of our Best Body Countdown meals take an average of 30 minutes to prepare from start to finish. Simple meals that take less than 30 minutes will have the Easy Meal icon. You may want to cluster all the easy meals on weeks that you are especially busy. Since many of the easy meals are perfect for "Lunch Leftovers," you can get even more mileage out of your brief kitchen time.

Many of the recipes are quick and easy, but we only use the Easy Meal
icon if the entire meal can be prepared simply in less than 30 minutes.

Pricey Meal

Over the course of 52 days, if your grocery budget allows for it, these occasional Pricey Meals provide a nice variety. Though not likely cost prohibitive, the ingredients for these meals do amount to slightly more than the others. While focusing on reaching Your Best Body, cutting back on dining out helps to allocate dollars for these special-occasion meals consumed at home where bottomless bread baskets and endless drink refills aren't warring against Best-Body progress.

Quicker-Fix

Most of our recipes are made from whole foods that require a small amount of preparation or chopping. However, we know that for some people, time and convenience are paramount, even if it costs more. Many of our recipes offer a Countdown Quicker-Fix to alert you to methods and convenience items that will save you time for that particular recipe. Look for the Quicker-Fix icon (instead of the golden arches) during seasons when every five minutes in your schedule counts.

Club Favorite

When I host the 52-day Best Body Countdown each New Year and fall, participants from all over the US join together for accountability, camaraderie, and my expert support through the Best Body Club private Facebook group. Best Body Club members have raved about their favorite recipes and want you to know which ones they like most: look for the Club Favorite icon. And, by the way, you are invited to join the Best Body Club, too. Anyone who plans to be lifelong-lean will need support somewhere along the way, so be sure to check out bestbodyin52.com.

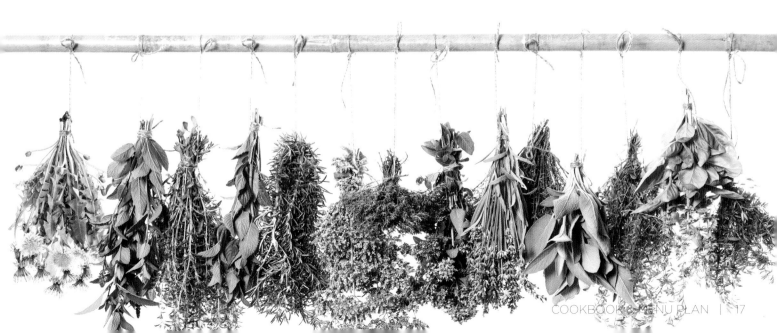

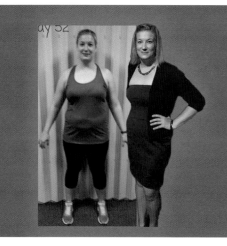

"52 days later ... This is something that I can do the rest of my life. I have new meals I like and I'm prepping and planning!."

—DENISE, 31

Be on the lookout for these terms:

Plate Plan Choices: portion out your meals using our Best Body Countdown Meal Measure tool, and our plate graphic and serving size guide

Best Body Beverages: recipes for smoothies and for flavored water using the Best Body Countdown Infuser bottle to give water an appealing zing

Best Body Breakfast: recipes you can rotate among your current healthy breakfasts

Strong Snack: suggestions and recipes for your pre-determined mid-day snack

Strategic Splurges: we suggest you plan your splurges in advance (3 or less per week recommended)

Tools

Our dietitian-approved recommendations for the upcoming 52-days:

- my **Countdown to Your Best Body Success Journal**
- Meal Measure or divided plate
- infuser water bottle
- garlic press
- silicone garlic peeler
- meat thermometer
- food processor or blender
- microplane zester
- sharp knives
- zip-top freezer storage bags
- pre-portioned snack cups for portion control
- adequate freezer space for buying healthy items on sale in bulk and for freezing
- double batches of healthy meals on hand in the freezer
- accountability partner and/or group support during the 52-day Best Body Countdown
- charts in the appendix, or the interactive download version of the same (bestbodyin52.com)
- video clips and blogs on the website: sign up for email updates!
- text @mybestbody to 81010 to get occasional text updates and new recipes

"Kitchen Clean-Up"

If you can say YES to these, GREAT!
- ❏ Are most of your foods perishable?
- ❏ Do you have at least 3 rainbow colors of fresh fruit?
- ❏ Do you have veggies in at least 3 colors?
- ❏ Do you have any beans without sodium added?
- ❏ Do you have fish filets (frozen or fresh), or canned tuna or salmon?
- ❏ Are your meats lean cuts (skinless poultry, loin or round cuts for beef and pork, or >90% lean ground beef)?
- ❏ Are your dressings low or reduced fat?
- ❏ Are your cheeses low or reduced fat?
- ❏ Does your milk say Fat-Free (skim) or Reduced Fat (1%) on it (or your non-dairy alternative)?
- ❏ Are there any ready-to-serve healthy homemade leftovers in your freezer?
- ❏ Is there a tidy table where you can eat mindfully and without distraction?
- ❏ Do you have more whole grains than refined grains? Such as:
  - ❏ Brown rice
  - ❏ Oats
  - ❏ Whole grain bread or pita
  - ❏ Whole grain crackers/crisp-breads
  - ❏ Whole grain cereal
  - ❏ Whole grain pasta

14

- ❏ If I stopped by right now and looked in your pantry and fridge would I say "You are all set to reach Your Best Body!"?

If you answer YES to most of the following, it's time for a kitchen make-over!
- ❏ Are most of the items in your kitchen boxed or canned?
- ❏ Do the grains come with seasoning packets? (ex: Rice a Roni, Hamburger Helper)
- ❏ On the labels of your cereals and snacks, are added sugars listed as main ingredients (one of the first 3-5 listed)?
- ❏ Are many of your foods artificially flavored and colored?
- ❏ Are there foods that make your fingers feel greasy after eating?
- ❏ Do the ingredient lists include hydrogenated oils?
- ❏ Are there tempting snacks or sweets in plain view, or at your eye-level in the pantry or refrigerator?
- ❏ What about heavily processed or fatty meats like hot dogs, sausage, salami or bologna?
- ❏ Is salt the first ingredient of most of your spices/seasonings?
- ❏ Is your eating space one that directs your mind elsewhere while eating? (for example, cluttered with paperwork, or set up in front of the TV)

Chart from the *Countdown to Your Best Body Success Journal*, page 14

Shopping Staples

FRESH PRODUCE (ALL!)

- ☑ Salad greens
- ☑ Bagged rainbow slaw (also called California slaw or broccoli slaw)
- ☑ Garlic (fresh, in the tube or minced)
- ☑ Onions (onions are storage produce and last a long time in the crisper drawer)
- ☑ Carrots (carrots last a long time in the refrigerator)
- ☑ Apples (apples keep well in the crisper drawer)
- ☑ Seasonal farmer's market specials

LEAN MEATS

- ☑ Fish
- ☑ Chicken and turkey breast
- ☑ Lean pork and beef (loin or round cuts)
- ☑ Canned tuna and salmon

WHOLE GRAINS, CEREALS, AND BEANS

- ☑ Canned reduced-sodium beans and bagged dry beans (black, pinto, navy, kidney, etc.)
- ☑ Whole grains (brown rice, whole-wheat pasta, barley, quinoa, old-fashioned or steel cut oats, etc.)
- ☑ Whole-grain pitas
- ☑ Ezekiel cinnamon-raisin English muffins

LOW-SODIUM CANNED GOODS AND DRIED FRUITS

- ☑ No-salt-added canned tomatoes (diced, stewed, and with green chilis)

- ☑ Reduced-sodium and unsalted stock or broth (chicken, vegetable, beef)

- ☑ Raisins (golden and purple)

DAIRY, EGGS, AND FROZEN FOODS

- ☑ Milk (1% or nonfat), plain soymilk or almond milk

- ☑ Eggs

- ☑ Butter or trans-fat-free spread

- ☑ Greek yogurt (plain, nonfat)

- ☑ Frozen fruit (blueberries, strawberries, blackberries, peaches)

- ☑ Frozen vegetables (stir-fry blends, mirepoix, chopped onions and peppers)

- ☑ Frozen chicken or fish (non-breaded)

MISCELLANEOUS

- ☑ Spice blends (Mrs. Dash salt-free seasonings, Jane's Krazy Mixed-Up Salt, Cavendar's Greek seasoning, grill seasonings, Italian seasoning, etc.)

- ☑ Healthy oil (canola oil, extra-virgin olive oil, canola oil cooking spray)

- ☑ Dressings such as Newman's Own Balsamic Vinegar and Bolthouse Farms Greek Yogurt Dressing

- ☑ Nuts and nut butter such as peanut butter or almond butter

Tips

THE PERFECT PLATE

Our recipes all have a nutrient breakdown at the bottom to help you learn what you are putting on your plate. We are not expecting you to count out every single gram of food from your day, but we do want you to be aware of how best to set up your meals. If your plate is set up properly, it generally translates into the appropriate nutrition numbers. The Plate Plan choices correlate with the Diabetes Exchange List established by the American Diabetes Association, as do the serving sizes in Appendix A.

When planning your lunch and dinner, always start with the bottom part of your plate, thinking of it as a big smile: happy because it's full of low-calorie, fiber-rich, disease-fighting vegetables. Cheesy, but memorable, right? Who would want a sad plate? This introduction will guide you as to what comprises a "Best Body Breakfast" and a "Strong Snack," too. I generally recommend fruit be served at those times, but it could also share the "smile" space on your plate, as long as vegetables are the priority.

Next, divide the top half of your plate into two quarters. In our recipes, if you see "3 lean meats" under the Nutrient Breakdown's Plate Plan choices, for example, that means that recipe provides about 3 ounces of lean meat to go in that quarter section of your plate. The other quarter of your plat should be starches, such as dried beans, whole grains, or starchy vegetables. (What if you want all three at once? Sure! Just know they have a pretty cozy "quarter" to share). Include a thumb-tip sized serving of fat, and your plate is set up for success.

CARBS AND SUGAR

When carbohydrates overflow out of this quarter of the plate is when they become problematic. Though people tend to fear carbs, typically the carbohydrate found in one quarter of their plate at planned meals is not the weight-gain culprit it gets made out to be. Now, carbs do deserve credit for belly fat and beyond when they come in the form of endless refills of chips, hot bread, and fries at restaurants, or desserts and caloric drinks. Limiting added sugar is essential during the Countdown. Though this adjustment can be tough at first, most actually notice a reduction in constant sugar cravings once they begin to limit their intake, not to mention a reduction in accumulating fat tissue.

Visualize your food fitting into the compartmentalized plate pictured. Consider using a plate divided into sections such as the Meal Measure that comes with my Best Body Countdown program or the divided plates you can get at your grocery store (or visit preciseportions.com for china options such as the one pictured here).

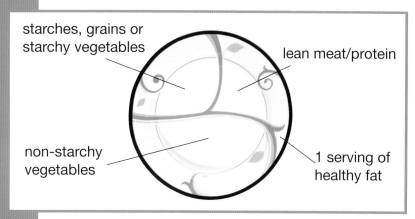

starches, grains or starchy vegetables

lean meat/protein

non-starchy vegetables

1 serving of healthy fat

Image from the *Countdown to Your Best Body Success Journal*, page 46

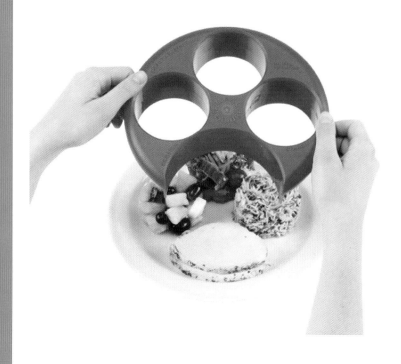

Each person reading this cookbook has his or her own unique nutrition needs. For some of you, these compartments will pile high, and for others less fuel is required. The serving sizes recommended in our recipes are average for most healthy adults, and are based on the balance suggested in the Countdown's guidelines for breakfast, lunch, and "Strong Snack," in addition to dinner. You may adjust the portions to meet your personal nutrition needs based on your activity level and lean mass. Additionally, you may want to consult a registered dietitian nutritionist to help you to individualize the serving sizes of the recipes based on your calculated calorie needs.

> "Your fuel needs (that is, your caloric needs), will depend on the size of your 'engine' (your lean body mass), and how much time you spend 'on the road' (moving and exercising)."

To get an idea about how much to put in each of the sections of the plate just described, refer to the "SmartCar vs. Expedition" analogy on page 25 in the *Countdown to Your Best Body Success Journal*

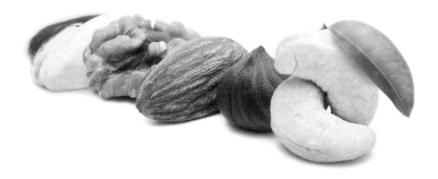

Start-Up Set-Up

We understand that your week may be busy, and if you are prioritizing exercise, that could be an added time commitment for you. You will need some strategy to make it all work. Setting aside about an hour to do some of the suggestions below when you have time on the weekend or at the beginning of your week will make all the difference.

> "One cannot think well, love well, sleep well, if one has not dined well."
>
> —VIRGINIA WOOLF

- Boil a half a dozen eggs to keep handy for use in quick breakfasts, lunches or "Strong Snacks."

- If you need quick ready-to-serve breakfasts for the week, choose from the "Best Body Breakfast" recipes offered in this cookbook and prepare in advance/freeze.

- Make sure you have some ready-to-eat vegetables and fruits available, whether you prep them during your pre-prep hour, or buy them cut and washed.

- Using our Staples List, prepare your grocery list for the week (see Appendix B to customize and make copies, or type it into the interactive grocery list you can download from bestbodyin52.com).

- If you like to have soup for lunches, drop a variety of frozen veggies, a can of diced tomatoes with chilies (such as Ro-tel), desired seasonings, and a couple of chicken breasts into a slow cooker with reduced-sodium broth in the morning on low heat. It will be ready for dinner that evening, and to warm up for lunches during the next few days of the week, even if you only have 5 minutes!

- Whenever you grill or cook lean meat, make extra for the upcoming days' salads, soups, and recipe ingredients.

- If you have the grill fired up, fill a grill basket with the vegetables you have on hand and you'll have delicious roasted veggies to add to any meal for the next few days.

- Start a slow cooker full of water on low and add 2 pounds of any dried beans you like: most take about 6 hours to cook. Drain and rinse well, allowing beans to cool. Set some aside for the upcoming week's salads, soups or sides and freeze the rest.

- Prepare grains or quinoa for meals in advance. Many of our recipes call for precooked grains. Having these ready at the start of the week, or in the freezer, makes dinner prep a snap (storing and freezing instructions to follow).

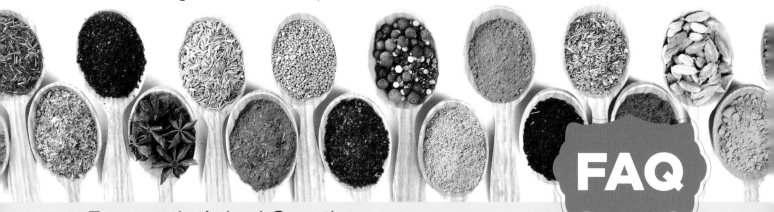

FAQ

Frequently Asked Question

What do you think about going gluten-free?

There are various reasons people avoid gluten, the protein in wheat, barley, and rye (and found in cross-contaminated oats). I have found that many who feel better on a gluten-free diet may feel just as good, without the challenges of going completely gluten-free, if they:

1. Trade out their refined grains for whole grains, choosing products with short ingredient lists and less preservatives.

2. Vary their grains/starches over the course of the day (intentionally eat grains besides wheat).

3. Make sure grain servings fit only on a quarter of their plate, or in the case of bread, limit it to 1-2 slices on their plate.

Excerpt from the *Countdown to Your Best Body Success Journal,* page 77-78

baked brown rice or barley

Total time: 20 minutes

This is a great way to cook both brown rice and barley. Not only does it turn out moist, but it is truly a timesaver! This recipe is plain (unseasoned), so you can use it in any recipe. It's ready fast, but without the extra cost and potential additives of quick-cook rice options.

Canola oil cooking spray

1 16-ounce bag of brown rice or barley

5 cups water (or 2½ cups reduced-sodium chicken broth and 2½ cups water)

1 tablespoon extra-virgin olive oil

¾ teaspoon salt

GROCERY LIST:
Brown rice or barley (16 ounces)
Reduced-sodium chicken broth (2½ cups)
Canola oil cooking spray
Extra-virgin olive oil
Salt
Flavor add-ins, as desired

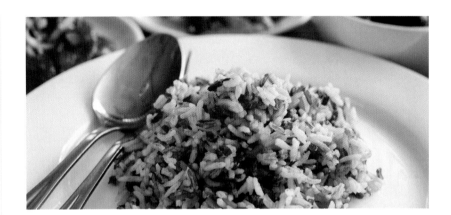

1. Preheat the oven to 375°F. Spray a 9x13-inch baking dish with cooking spray and add brown rice.

2. Bring the water to a boil, add oil and salt, and pour the mixture over the rice. Stir to combine, cover tightly with heavy-duty aluminum foil and bake for 60 minutes.

3. Once done, remove aluminum foil and fluff rice with a fork. Cover with a clean kitchen towel for 5 minutes. Uncover for another 5 minutes, then fluff with a fork and serve or freeze as desired.

Yield: 10 cups or 30 servings
(serving size: ¹/₃ cup)

Nutrient Breakdown:
for brown rice (barley):

Calories 60

Fat 1g

Cholesterol 5mg

Sodium 60mg

Carbohydrate 12g

Fiber 1g (2g)

Protein 1g (2g)

Plate Plan choices:
1 starch

precooked quinoa

Quinoa can be cooked ahead of time and stored 3–5 days in the refrigerator or for 2 months in the freezer.

INGREDIENTS AND GROCERY LIST:

Plain quinoa

Reduced-sodium chicken broth

Flavor add-ins as desired

1. Cook unflavored quinoa ahead by following the directions on the package, except use half water and half reduced-sodium chicken broth to cook the quinoa.

2. Once cooked, allow the quinoa to cool.

Nutrient Breakdown:
(serving size: 1/3 cup cooked)

Calories 70

Fat 1g

Sodium 35mg

Carbohydrate 13g

Fiber 2g

Protein 3g

Plate Plan choices:
1 starch

flavor add-in suggestions:

Sautéed onions, shallots, celery, bell pepper, mushrooms, or garlic

Citrus zest, toasted nuts, or dried fruits

Examples:

lemon zest + parsley + toasted almonds

orange zest + cumin + cilantro

storing and freezing

To store precooked grains, quinoa or prepared dried beans, place 1½–2-cup portions into sandwich bags (with date noted), removing the air and flattening the contents. Then place the filled bags in a gallon-sized plastic zip-top freezer bag. Freeze for up to 2 months. To use, simply remove from the sandwich bag and transfer the grain/beans to a microwave-safe bowl, cover with a damp paper towel, and microwave for 1–2 minutes, stirring halfway through warming time. Add an additional minute or two if necessary.

READ THE RECIPE

It is important to read the entire recipe prior to beginning to cook. You don't want to be an hour away from meal time only to learn you were supposed to refrigerate something for a couple of hours or marinate overnight.

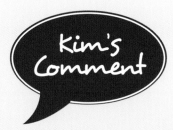

GATHER INGREDIENTS FIRST

Practice *mise en place*: pronounced [MEEZ ahn plahs]. This is a French term that literally translates to "set in place." It is a practice that professional chefs use before they begin cooking, and it is a real time saver for the home cook as well.

Gathering your ingredients together before you begin to cook allows you to verify that you have the ingredients you need. It also allows the cooking process to proceed smoothly without interruption. Think of it like taking a shower: all of what you need to get clean is already in the shower, so there is no need to get out to get the soap, shampoo, and conditioner. The same principle applies to cooking: if all your ingredients are gathered and ready, the process flows more efficiently.

GET YOUR PAN JUST RIGHT

Let your pan and oil or butter get hot before adding ingredients. A hot pan is essential for sautéing veggies or creating a great crust on meat, fish, and poultry. It also helps prevent food from sticking. Take care that it doesn't get too hot. No smoking oil, please!

Avoid over-crowding the pan. Food releases moisture as it's cooked, so leave room for the steam to escape and let the food brown. The brown crusty bits are critical for flavor, particularly with lower-fat cooking. Cook in batches if necessary.

Best Body Breakfast

Is breakfast really the most important meal of the day? Absolutely! People who skip breakfast have a hard time meeting their fiber needs, often overeat later in the day or evening, and are not well fueled for an active day (not to mention they might have a bit of a foggy brain). Those who want to be at their best need to fuel up well for their day. One of the five essentials of the Best Body Countdown is to eat three balanced meals (and a "Strong Snack") daily.

I often hear, "I don't have time for breakfast." Now, Kim and I can't help you get up 5–10 minutes earlier to prioritize breakfast, but we do have some suggestions for quick breakfasts. At some point, most people tire of feeling sluggish, foggy, and "belly heavy" and give breakfast a try.

For those who feel they can't stomach breakfast in the early morning or have a hard time eating first thing related to their morning workout timing, try my *breakfast block* strategy: meet the **Best Body Breakfast** guidelines within 4 hours of waking up, even if it's not all once.

A **Best Body Breakfast** meets the following criteria to start your day off strong:

☑ At least 7–10 grams fiber from 1–3 grain servings (depending on your fuel needs and activity level), and 1 fruit serving*

☑ 15–30 grams of protein (from all of the food groups combined over the *breakfast block*)

☑ 300–500 mg calcium (typically found in 1 dairy serving, noted below):
- skim or 1% milk or yogurt (1 cup)
- reduced-fat cheese (1.5 ounces)
- low-fat cottage cheese (¼ cup)

- a dairy alternative fortified with calcium such as soy milk, rice milk, almond milk, or orange juice (see product label for calcium quantity)

- or a 300–500 mg calcium supplement

☑ 5–15 grams of fat, ideally from a small serving of nuts

*Check out Appendix A for serving sizes of common foods, and Appendix F for a list of foods containing fiber.

Breakfast suggestions that take less than 5 minutes to prepare and about 5 minutes to eat:

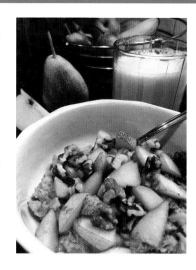

old fashioned oatmeal

Cover ¼ cup old-fashioned rolled oats with water and microwave for 3 minutes on high in a deep, microwave-safe bowl. While it cooks, dice up a ripe pear (or a small apple), and pour a glass of milk. Add the pear, a tablespoon of raisins and a dash of cinnamon. You'll be surprised at how you don't really miss the sugar like you'd expect.

english muffin

Spread almond butter over an Ezekiel cinnamon-raisin English muffin and serve with a glass of milk.

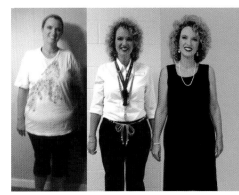

"Breakfast is a non-negotiable as it relates to my success in maintaining my weight loss.

—SONYA, 49

basic eggs and toast

Sprinkle eggs with reduced fat cheese and serve with whole-grain toast and a piece of fruit.

Also, many of the breakfast recipes that follow can be prepared in advance so that they don't take much time from your morning. Some just need to be quickly toasted, warmed or defrosted. Shake recipes follow as well - simply requiring a moment in the blender before you take them on your way out the door on those mornings you don't have time to sit down to eat.

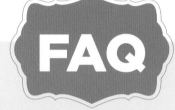

Frequently Asked Question

Why is the sugar content in yogurt so high?

Yogurt is tricky because the "sugars" on the label can be from both naturally occurring sugars (the milk sugar, lactose, and the fruit sugar, fructose) as well as added sugars. Sugar that naturally occurs in milk or fruit is not considered "added" sugar, therefore does not count towards the sugar-gram totals recommended during the Best Body Countdown. Regardless, moderation is always key! Greek yogurt has more protein to hold you over to your next meal, and naturally less sugar. Plus, those who are lactose intolerant can tolerate small amounts of Greek yogurt better. Plain, nonfat Greek yogurt is our yogurt of choice for our recipes such as the Raspberry Power Parfait on page 36.

The following breakfast recipes are suitable to be made in advance, so you can grab a quick breakfast in the morning if needed.

apricot baked oatmeal

Hands-on time: 20 minutes
Total time: 60 minutes (includes oven time)

This is delicious! It is the earthiness of the oats and the slight sweetness of the banana that make this a tasty grab-and-go breakfast.

suggested side: berries and milk

Canola oil cooking spray

2½ cups dry rolled oats

1 teaspoon baking powder

1 teaspoon cinnamon

1¾ cups milk

2 large bananas, mashed

2 eggs

¾ cup nonfat, plain Greek yogurt

3 tablespoons chia seeds

¾ teaspoon almond extract

10 dried apricot halves, chopped

½ cup slivered almonds

GROCERY LIST:

Bananas (2 large)

Rolled oats (2½ cups)

Slivered almonds (½ cup)

Chia seeds (3 tablespoons)

Dried apricot halves (10 halves)

Milk (1¾ cup + suggested side)

Plain, nonfat Greek yogurt (¾ cup)

Eggs (2)

Baking powder

Cinnamon

Almond extract

Canola oil cooking spray

Berries (suggested side)

Kim's Comment

This is wonderful baked on a week-end and then served throughout the week. I have used it as a grab-and-go breakfast with much success.

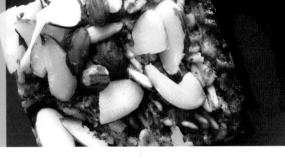

1. Preheat oven to 350°F. Spray an 8x8-inch pan with cooking spray and set aside.

2. In a large bowl, whisk together the oats, baking powder and cinnamon. In a medium bowl, combine the milk, banana, eggs, yogurt, chia seeds and extract. Stir to combine. Add the milk mixture to the oats and stir until thoroughly combined. Fold in the apricots. Pour the mixture into the prepared dish and bake for 10 minutes. Add almonds and bake for 30–35 additional minutes until done. Allow it to cool before cutting into 12 pieces.

Yield: 6 servings
(serving size: 2 pieces)

Nutrient Breakdown:
Calories 330

Fat 11g (2g saturated fat)

Cholesterol 65mg

Sodium 170mg

Carbohydrate 45g

Fiber 8g

Protein 15g

Plate Plan Choices: 1½ starches, 1 fruit, ½ milk, 1 protein, 1 fat

To make this an approved Best Body Breakfast, serve one of the following two ways:

Option 1: 2 slices (1 serving), plus ½ cup of milk

Option 2: 1 slice (½ serving), plus 1 cup berries (or other high-fiber fruit) plus 1 cup milk

sweet potato oat pancakes

Full of flavor and protein, perfect to get your day started on the right track. Pancakes are great to make on the weekend and freeze or refrigerate for use during the week. If you make a double batch, you'll use the whole sweet potato and have enough for a busy morning: we recommend it!

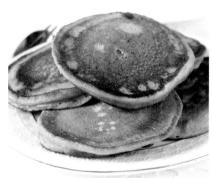

suggested toppings:
apple-chia jam or chia peanut butter

Total time: 25 minutes

1 sweet potato (scrubbed clean) or ½ cup pureed pumpkin

1½ cup dry rolled oats

3 eggs

½ cup low-fat cottage cheese or plain, nonfat Greek yogurt

¼–½ cup nonfat or 1% milk

1½ teaspoon baking powder

⅛ teaspoon salt

1 teaspoon cinnamon

1 teaspoon vanilla

Canola oil cooking spray

Nutmeg (optional garnish)

1. Carefully pierce the sweet potato skin 5–6 times and microwave for 5–8 minutes, rotating after a few minutes. Once the potato is cooked, slice it in half and allow to cool for a couple minutes. Scoop the flesh out of the peel and mash. Tip: hold the potato with an oven mitt while scooping out the flesh to avoid getting burned.

2. Add ½ cup of mashed sweet potato and remaining ingredients to a blender. Blend until smooth. You may need to add a little more fluid (milk or water) if your batter is thick.

3. Heat a nonstick skillet or griddle on medium-low heat (300–350°F). Spray with cooking spray. For each pancake, pour ¼ cup of batter onto griddle or skillet. Allow the pancakes to bubble. Flip to cook on the second side until golden brown. Serve with Apple-Chia Jam or Chia Peanut Butter.

Yield: 4 servings
(serving size: 3 pancakes)

Nutrient Breakdown:
Calories 230

Fat 6g (1.5g saturated fat)

Cholesterol 135mg

Sodium 230mg

Carbohydrate 31g

Fiber 4g

Protein 13g

Plate Plan choices:
2 starches, ½ fat, 1 lean meat

GROCERY LIST:
Sweet potato (1) or 1 can pureed pumpkin

Rolled oats (1½ cups)

Eggs (3)

Low-fat cottage cheese or plain, nonfat Greek yogurt (½ cup)

Nonfat or 1% milk (½ cup)

Baking powder

Salt

Cinnamon

Vanilla

Nutmeg (optional garnish)

Canola oil cooking spray

GROCERY LIST:
for Apple Chia Jam (suggested topping)
Apple (1)

Apple juice (1 cup)
Suggestion: keep individual servings of juice on hand

Chia seeds (2 tablespoons)

GROCERY LIST:
for Peanut Butter Chia Spread (alternate suggested topping)

Peanut butter (¼ cup)

Chia seeds (3 tablespoons)

To make this an approved **Best Body Breakfast**, serve one of the two following ways:

 Serve with ¼ cup Apple-Chia Jam and a cup of milk

Apple-Chia Jam Recipe: Place 1 finely chopped or grated apple (peel on) in a medium saucepan with 1 cup apple juice and 2 tablespoons chia seeds. Cook over medium heat until the mixture boils and then reduce heat to simmer for 5 additional minutes until the fruit softens a little and the mixture thickens. Remove from heat and serve on pancakes. We know it doesn't look anything like syrup, but you've got to try it: it's delicious! The jam will last about a week in the refrigerator and can be made with other fruits such as strawberries and blueberries. This is also great as a yogurt topping.

 Serve with Chia Peanut Butter and a cup of milk

Chia Peanut Butter Recipe: Place ¼ cup peanut butter in a microwave-safe bowl and microwave for 20 seconds. Stir in 3 tablespoons of chia seeds. Divide mixture among 4 servings of pancakes.

Nutrient Breakdown with jam:
Calories 290, Fat 7.5g, Carbohydrate 41g, Fiber 8g, Protein 14g

Nutrient Breakdown with jam and milk
(suggested): Calories 370, Fat 7.5g, Carbohydrate 53g, Fiber 8g, Protein 22g

Nutrient Breakdown with Chia Peanut Butter: Calories 370, Fat 16g, Carbohydrate 38g, Fiber 8g, Protein 18g

Nutrient Breakdown with Chia Peanut Butter and milk: Calories 450, Fat 16g, Carbohydrate 50g, Fiber 8g, Protein 26g

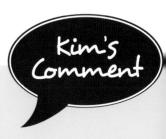

Kim's Comment

Chia seeds, while small, pack a big fiber punch. While we do not believe in being a slave to nutrition numbers, we do think it is critical to start each day with a good dose of fiber. Not only are chia seeds a great plant source of omega-3 fatty acids, but they also provide 4 grams of fiber per tablespoon.

raspberry power parfait

Total time: 10 minutes + refrigerator time (overnight if desired)

Easy Meal

It's ideal to prepare this the night before serving. This is as close to perfect as a breakfast can get: ready to serve when you wake up, calcium, fiber and protein rich, no sugar added, and holds you over strong from breakfast until lunch! You may want to double or triple the recipe, as this can be refrigerated up to 5 days and portioned into mason jars to take on the go.

½ cup plain soymilk

1 tablespoon ground flaxseed (or flaxseed meal)

1 tablespoon chia seeds

½ cup plain, nonfat Greek yogurt

1 teaspoon vanilla extract

¼ cup old-fashioned oats

¾ cup raspberries, frozen or fresh

Cinnamon, to taste

GROCERY LIST:

Raspberries, frozen or fresh (¾ cup)

Old-fashioned oats (¼ cup)

Ground flaxseeds or flaxseed meal

Chia seeds

Plain soymilk or other unsweetened milk (½ cup)

Plain, nonfat Greek yogurt (½ cup)

Vanilla extract

Cinnamon

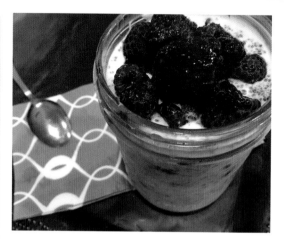

Yield: 1 serving
(serving size: 1 large serving without honey or granola)

Nutrient Breakdown:
Calories 333
Fat 9.75g (0.75g saturated fat)
Carbohydrate 43.5g
Fiber 15.5g
Protein 15g

Plate Plan choices:
1 fruit, 1 milk, 1 starch,
1 lean meat, 1 fat

1. In a bowl or a jar that has a lid, put all ingredients in the order they are listed above, except the berries.
2. Stir to combine well.
3. Add raspberries and gently mix until throughout. This can be eaten right away or allowed to thicken overnight. Serve with cinnamon, if desired.

"I make this at the beginning of the week for me and my husband and put it in snap-top containers to grab in the mornings. It's a great way to start the day."
—MICHELLE, 35

If you need to sweeten this tart treat, add ½ teaspoon of honey when it's time to serve. Or, if you like it sweet and crunchy, add a tablespoon or two of granola. If you prefer a smooth consistency, try oat bran instead of rolled oats. Any berries will work well if raspberries aren't on hand. My youngest child and I make this every Sunday night at my house in large glass bowl and keep it handy for ready-made **Best Body Breakfasts** and **Strong Snacks** all week!

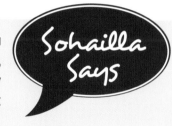

Sohailla Says

quiche breakfast to-go

Hands-on time: 20–25 minutes
Total time: 20–25 minutes

Easy Meal

These have a great flavor and one recipe makes several days' worth of grab-and-go breakfasts. Keep some in the refrigerator for this week and freeze the rest for next week or beyond.

Canola oil cooking spray

5 Flatout Foldits

6 eggs

3 egg whites

½ cup reduced-fat sharp cheddar cheese

2 cloves garlic, minced

½ cup finely diced onion

4 cups chopped raw spinach (lightly packed)

2 plum tomatoes, chopped (~¾ cup)

½ teaspoon Cavender's Greek seasoning or seasoning blend of choice

GROCERY LIST:

Baby spinach (4 cups)

Plum or Roma tomatoes (2)

Garlic cloves (2)

Onion (1 medium)

Flatout Foldit flatbreads (5)

Eggs (9)

Reduced-fat sharp cheddar (½ cup)

Cavender's Greek seasoning or seasoning of choice

Canola oil cooking spray

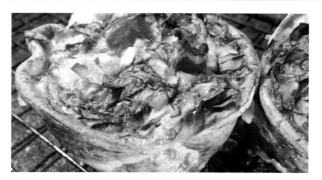

1. Preheat the oven to 375°F and spray 10 muffin cups with non-stick cooking spray. Cut the flatbreads in half (widthwise) and press them into the muffin cups. Make sure to press the flatbread into the cups so that the bottom of the cup is covered with flatbread and overlap the edges of the flatbread around the sides of the cup, pressing them together (this will decrease the likelihood of the egg mixture leaking out).

2. In a large bowl, whisk the eggs until well combined. Add in the remaining ingredients and mix.

3. Carefully fill each Flatout with the egg mixture (just under ½ cup). Bake for 20–25 minutes or until done in the center.

Yield:
10 servings
(serving size: 1 muffin)

Nutrient Breakdown:
Calories 180

Fat 7g (2.5g saturated fat)

Cholesterol 180mg

Sodium 400mg

Carbohydrate 14g

Fiber 5g

Protein 18g

Plate Plan choices:
1 starch, 1 medium-fat meat/protein, 1 vegetable

These will freeze well. Simply wrap in plastic or foil and place in a freezer bag. You can literally grab and go after a quick minute on defrost in the microwave! We suggest adding a piece of fruit and a cup of milk.

healthy harvest muffins

With 4 grams of protein, 4 grams of healthy fat, and 4 grams of fiber, these will give you great "holding power." They freeze well and take some chopping effort, so you may as well make a double batch. When ready to eat, simply use the microwave and defrost for about a minute for 1 muffin, and it comes out perfectly (best if served warm)!

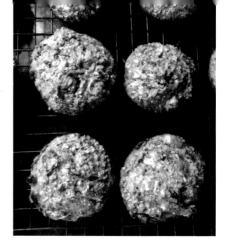

Hands-on time: 25 minutes   Total time: 50 minutes

Canola oil cooking spray

1 cup Bob's Red Mill 7-grain cereal with flax (or similar mix)

¾ cup + 2 tablespoons white whole-wheat flour

1 tablespoon baking powder

2 teaspoons cinnamon

2 over-ripe bananas, mashed

1 large zucchini, shredded

1½ cups shredded carrot

1 large apple (skin on), finely chopped

½ cup nonfat milk

2 eggs

½ cup plain, nonfat Greek yogurt

2 teaspoons vanilla

1 cup golden raisins

¼ cup chia seeds

½ cup walnuts or pecans, finely chopped

1. Preheat oven to 400°F.
2. Line 18 muffin tins with paper liners or spray muffin tins with cooking spray.
3. In a large bowl, whisk the dry ingredients together (multi-grain cereal through cinnamon).
4. In a medium bowl, mix the wet ingredients together (banana through vanilla).
5. Make a well in the flour mixture and pour the wet ingredients into the center of the well.
6. Mix batter until just combined. Fold in raisins, chia seeds and nuts. The batter will be thick.
7. Spoon into muffin cups (~¼ cup batter per muffin).
8. Bake 20–25 minutes or until golden brown. They may still be a bit gooey in the middle, so check to see if they need a few more minutes.

GROCERY LIST:

Bananas (2 over-ripe)

Zucchini (1 large)

Carrots (1½ cups shredded)

Apple (1 large)

Bob's Red Mill (or similar) 7-grain cereal with flax (1 cup)

Chia seeds

Milk (½ cup)

Eggs (2)

Plain, nonfat Greek yogurt (½ cup)

Walnuts or Pecans (½ cup)

White whole-wheat flour (¾ cup plus 2 tablespoons)

Golden raisins (1 cup)

Baking powder

Cinnamon

Vanilla

Yield:
18 muffins

Nutrient Breakdown:
(serving size: 1 muffin)

Calories 140

Fat 4g (0.5 g saturated fat)

Cholesterol 20mg

Sodium 150mg

Carbohydrate 23g

Fiber 4g

Protein 4g

Plate Plan choices:
½ starch, 1 fruit, ½ protein, 1 fat

Strategic Splurges

As a general rule, the Best Body Countdown guidelines suggest three Strategic Splurges per week. How a splurge is defined is up to you. This means you decide in advance what it will be and set yourself up to savor each bite or sip, mindful of your portion-sizes. Examples include fried foods or chips, sweets, caloric beverages, snack foods, chocolate, alcoholic beverages, or pizza. Keep in mind that eating out pretty much will count as your Strategic Splurge even if you don't choose especially rich food due to the preparation methods and portion sizes typically served at restaurants.

On a very special occasion, you may have all three splurges for the week in one day, and sometimes you may want to have a really tiny splurge two days in a row that just adds up to one of your three. The point is that you are strategic and mindful, leaving no room for careless ("did I eat that?") munching, binging, or regret-based determinations.

Check out the **Countdown to Your Best Body Success Journal** for more information about alcohol and other splurges.

> **"** It's easy to say 'no!' when there's a
>
> deeper 'yes!' burning inside."
>
> —STEPHEN COVEY

Sweet-Tooth Satisfiers

CREAMY:

Add about 60 Ghirardelli mini semi-sweet chocolate baking chips (that's about 2 tablespoons, just 35 calories and 4 grams of added sugar) to plain Greek yogurt with ¾ cup of chopped strawberries.

CRUNCHY:

If it's a cookie you're after, think "small is better than not at all" and know you'll have to bump a starch plus a fat serving to make room in your day for two Oreo-sized cookies.

HOT:

One packet of Swiss Miss 25-calorie hot chocolate plus 2 tablespoons mini-marshmallows (totaling 45 calories, 4g added sugar)

COLD:

Frozen blueberries or raspberries (¾ cup = 1 fruit serving, 0g added sugar)

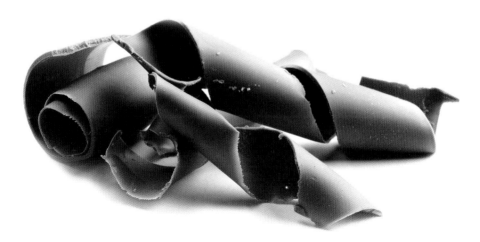

Coffee and Cream Shake

¼ cup Edy's Slow Churned French Silk Ice Cream, 3 ounces chilled black coffee, 3 ounces unsweetened almond milk, cinnamon to taste.

1. Combine the first 3 ingredients with ½ cup of ice in a blender and process until frothy.

2. Sprinkle with cinnamon and serve immediately.

Nutrient Breakdown: Calories 78, Fat 5g, Carb 11g, Fiber 0g, Protein 3g, Sodium 60g, Sugars 8g (about 6g of which is added sugar)

Sweet Protein Perfection

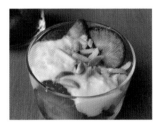

Sweet, quick and nutritious too! See page 108 for recipe.

CAKE-LIKE:

Strong Snack Mug Cake

In a small bowl, mix 1 large ripe mashed banana, 1 tablespoon of any nut butter, 1 egg, 2 teaspoons chopped walnuts, 3 level tablespoons cocoa powder, and 1 teaspoon honey. Pour into 2 small mugs. Microwave on high for 2 minutes (one mug at a time). Or, if you are sharing one large mug cake, microwave on high for 2½ minutes. Serve with 8 ounces of milk.

Nutrient Breakdown for 1 cake: Calories 200, Fat 9g, Carbohydrate 22g, Fiber 4g, Sodium 65mg, Protein 7g

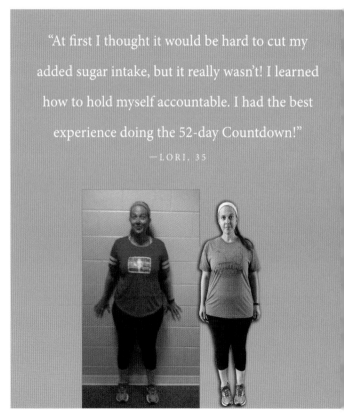

"At first I thought it would be hard to cut my added sugar intake, but it really wasn't! I learned how to hold myself accountable. I had the best experience doing the 52-day Countdown!"

—LORI, 35

pita pizza

Easy Meal

Perfect for a fun lunch or a super-quick dinner, and a whole round is about the same number of calories as just one slice of restaurant pizza! These are always a hit with kids, too!

4 whole-wheat pita rounds

¼ cup pizza sauce

1½ cup fresh baby spinach, chopped

2 teaspoons chopped fresh basil

1 cup shredded part-skim mozzarella cheese, divided

¼ cup chopped red onion

1 cup chopped tomato

1 cup chopped red bell pepper

1 2.25-ounce can sliced black olives

1 teaspoon dried oregano

24 pepperoni rounds, cut into quarters (about 6 per pizza)

GROCERY LIST:

Baby spinach (1 1/2 cups)

Fresh basil

Red onion (1 small)

Tomato (1 cup chopped)

Red bell pepper (1)

Whole-wheat pita rounds (4)

Pizza sauce (¼ cup)

Sliced black olives (2.25-ounce can)

Pepperoni rounds (24)

Part-skim mozzarella cheese (1 cup)

Dried oregano

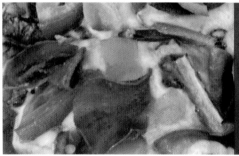

Pizza is another splurge that quickly gets people over their calorie budget for the day. If ordering pizza occasionally, have a big salad and think of pizza more as a "side." Or even better, try this recipe for both at once: pizza and veggies in each bite!

1. Preheat oven to 400°F. Place the pita rounds on a baking sheet and spoon 1 tablespoon of pizza sauce over each.

2. Evenly distribute the chopped spinach and basil over the pita rounds.

3. Spoon 2 tablespoons of cheese over each pita (about half of the cheese will be used here). Add the remaining toppings (onions through olives).

4. Sprinkle the remaining cheese and oregano over the pizzas and top with pepperoni.

5. Bake at 400°F for 7–10 minutes or until the cheese is bubbly and edges are beginning to brown.

Yield: 4 servings
(serving size: 1 pita pizza)

Nutrient Breakdown:
Calories 281

Fat 10g, (4g saturated fat)

Sodium 752mg

Carbohydrate 35g

Fiber 6g

Protein 16g

Plate Plan choices:
2 starches, 1 vegetable, 1½ medium fat meats, 1 fat

"These are a hit with my entire family!

The kids like to help add toppings.

They're easy to make and delicious!"

—DENA, 44

Strong Snacks

Choose one from each category in the following chart for what I consider a Strong Snack, or try some of the suggested recipes listed such as the Raspberry Power Parfait breakfast recipe or the upcoming Sunflower Seed Spread. Strategically schedule this snack at that time of the day where the hungry monster tries to make you frantic for food, despite the fact that your typical mealtime is a couple hours away. This Strong Snack combination typically ensures a minimum of 5 grams of protein and 3 grams of fiber, both of which meet your midday nutrition needs and help to hold you over gracefully until your final meal of the day. Choosing one item from each column will be about a 200–300 calorie snack. Because they are healthy choices, they won't really "spoil your supper." If you eat a little less at supper because you ate at healthy snack at 3:30 p.m., that's no loss. If you are especially active, you may need to have two Strong Snacks daily.

STRONG SNACK SUGGESTIONS:

Healthy Harvest Muffin

Sweet Protein Perfection

Avocado Salsa Topper

Watermelon Feta Salad

Klassic 3-seed Dr. Kracker
Crispbreads with cheese

Edamame

Sunflower Seed Spread

Monkey Shake

Raspberry Power Parfait

DAIRY OR ALTERNATIVE	FRUIT (LOOK FOR FIBER AND COLOR VARIETY!)	HEALTHY FAT (1 FAT SERVING= 50 CALORIES)
1 cup milk (fat free or 1%), or 1 cup soy milk, rice milk or almond milk	1/2 banana or any other fruit (see portion sizes in Appendix J)	pecans or walnuts: 4 halves (50 calories) or 8 halves (100 calories)
6-8 ounces of yogurt (go for Greek)	3/4 cup raspberries or any other berries	sunflower seeds (1 tbsp = 50 calories)
1/4 cup Fat Free or 1% cottage cheese	1 orange, or any other tennis-ball sized fruit	large olives - 8 black, 10 green (stuffed)
string cheese piece	1 medium apple, sliced	1-1/2 tsp peanut butter
milk with cereal noted to the right:	occasional cereal substitute: look for >3 grams of protein and >2 g fiber in a 15 gram carb portion (see label)	10 peanuts or 16 pistachios (50 calories) almonds or cashews 6 (50) or 12 (100)
1.5 ounce of reduced fat cheese	occasional substitute: 15 grams carb portion of whole grain crackers	2 tablespoons avocado (1/5th of an avocado)

Excerpt from the *Countdown to Your Best Body Success Journal,* page 59

sunflower seed spread

This recipe is always a hit! You should have seen the response when we did a taste test…
it's surprisingly delicious!

3 cups sunflower seeds (unsalted if available)

¾ cup lemon juice

¼ cup almond butter

3 garlic cloves

1–2 teaspoons fresh ginger, grated

1 teaspoon cumin

1 teaspoon salt

¼ teaspoon dried cayenne pepper, or to taste

1 cup kale

1 red bell pepper

1 cup sweet onion

1 cup fresh parsley stems removed

GROCERY LIST:

Garlic cloves (3 cloves)

Fresh ginger (2-inch piece)

Kale (1 cup)

Red bell pepper (1)

Sweet onion (1 cup chopped)

Parsley (1 cup)

Lemon juice (¾ cup)

Sunflower seeds, unsalted if available (3 cups)

Almond butter (¼ cup)

Cumin

Salt

Cayenne pepper

1. Grind sunflower seeds in a food processor. Transfer to a mixing bowl.

2. Combine the lemon juice, almond butter and spices in the food processor and process until mixed.

3. Add all of the vegetables and pulse. There should be little pieces and the color of all the veggies but not big chunks.

4. Combine the vegetable mixture with the ground sunflower seeds in the mixing bowl. Serve with cut fresh vegetables or spread on whole-grain crackers.

Yield: 32 2-tablespoon servings or 4 cups

Nutrient Breakdown:
Calories 80

Fat 6g (1g saturated fat)

Sodium 70mg

Carbohydrate 5g

Fiber 2g

Protein 3g

Plate Plan choices:
½ vegetable, ½ lean meat/protein, 1 fat

To make this a Best Body Countdown Strong Snack, serve with either:
Raw Veggies (cucumber, carrots, and red bell pepper)
Flatbread crackers and a cup of milk

To make this for lunch, serve rolled up in a whole-grain wrap with fresh spinach. Delish!

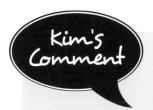

Kim's Comment

Unless you are taking it as an appetizer somewhere, this makes a bit much to eat at once, even if you love it like I do. The good news is that this gem of a recipe freezes well. I usually freeze it in small disposable plastic containers in ¼-cup portions. That way, I can just pull a container out and thaw it in the refrigerator when I need a quick snack later that day. Or, I might pull a couple containers out if I need an appetizer on the fly.

Best Body Beverages

FRESHLY INFUSED WATER RECIPES

Adequate water intake is critical to good health: one of the five Best Body Countdown essentials is to have four water bottles daily. While leading the Best Body Club Facebook page and reading participants' vents, I have come to realize just how many people are "water-haters." So, I've added a fabulous infuser bottle to my programs that helps minimize excuses and maximize hydration. Herb- or produce-infused water counts as REAL water and is a refreshing change from plain water.

When you take a look at these delightful infused water recipes, you can tell which one of us is the foodie and which one of us still has hip-high little ones at home tugging a leg in the kitchen. Kim is the "recipe fancy pants," and I tend to keep it simple in the kitchen, for this season anyway!

KIM'S INFUSED WATER FAVORITES:

Cucumber Mint Cooler:

Several thin slices of cucumber

A few sprigs of mint

Shake well and let sit for a while (preferably overnight) before enjoying.

This is so refreshing and makes a good pick-me-up mid-afternoon.

Orange Spritzer:

Fresh cut oranges (rinds removed)

Slice of lime (give it a slight squeeze into the water bottle)

Thinly sliced fresh ginger root (to get the most flavor, smash the peeled ginger a little)

If you like a bubbly beverage, you can add a dash of club soda after shaking well. This makes a really nice evening beverage to sip on in place of a cocktail or wine.

Take-me-to-Jamaica Punch:

Strawberries, sliced

Fresh-cut orange wedges
(wash rinds well)

Cantaloupe slices (rinds removed)

Shake well and let sit for a while (preferably overnight) before sipping. My favorite place in the world is Jamaica, and this is just the right blend to bring on the memories.

Easy Does It:

Peeled orange sections or fresh cut orange wedges (rinds removed)

Honestly, this is surprisingly perfect as-is after a quick shake of the infuser bottle.

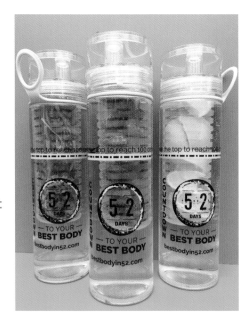

SMOOTHIES AND SHAKES

Monkey Shake

Place the following into your blender in this order:

1 cup milk

½ banana

½ cup ice

1 teaspoon cocoa

¼ cup vanilla Greek yogurt (or ¼ cup fat free cottage cheese)

1½ teaspoons natural creamy peanut butter

Blend on high until smooth.

Yield: 1 serving

Nutrient Breakdown (using 1% milk): Calories 259, Fat 8g, Carb 32g, Fiber 3g, Protein 17g

Monster Shake

Place into your blender in this order:

½ cup milk

½ cup peach low fat Greek yogurt

¼ cup 100% apple juice or grape juice

3 frozen peach wedges (or fresh)

½ cup ice, and a handful of baby spinach (about 1 cup of leaves), raw and washed.

Blend on high until smooth. Drink promptly.

Yield: 1 serving

Nutrient Breakdown (using 1% milk): Calories 196, Fat 2g, Carb 34g, Fiber 2g, Protein 12g

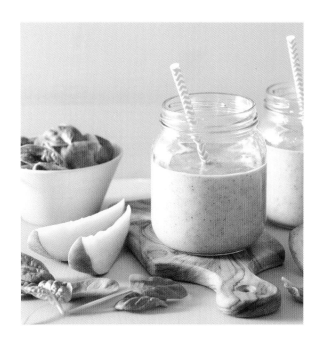

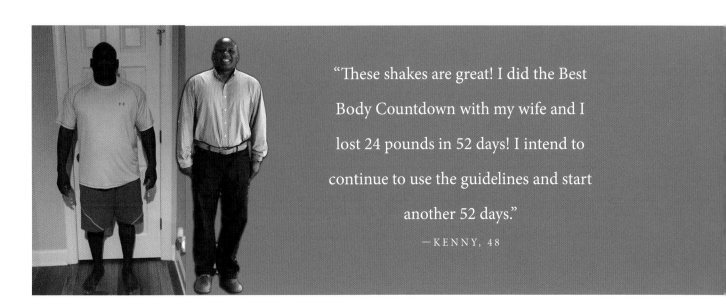

"These shakes are great! I did the Best Body Countdown with my wife and I lost 24 pounds in 52 days! I intend to continue to use the guidelines and start another 52 days."

—KENNY, 48

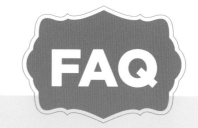

Frequently Asked Question:

"What about having a drink?"

How drinking alcohol impacts your health and weight is largely dependent on how much you have, and your overall calorie balance. First, let's define a standard alcoholic "drink:"

12 oz. of beer (0 added sugars)

5 oz. of wine (most have 1-5g sugars)

1.5 oz. or a "shot" of liquor (0 added sugars initially)

Moderate drinking is defined as up to one daily drink for a woman, and up to two for a man. Though moderate alcohol intake can be part of a healthy diet, our nation's obesity level is an indication of how difficult moderation is. In addition to the calories consumed in the beverage (including the mixers) and the way the body processes alcohol into fat tissue readily, drinking can impact the number of servings you choose to eat at that time, and can increase the risk of certain cancers. So, the question to ask yourself is, "Is it worth it?" If you decide it is, then mindfully savor each sip, having committed to your limit in advance.

Excerpt from the *Countdown to Your Best Body Success Journal,* page 42

Happy Half-a-Plate

Do you recall that half of your lunch and dinner plate should be thought of as a big smile—**happy** because it's full of healthy vegetables? Many people dread eating veggies, but in our experience, we've learned it's mostly because they haven't yet tried the preparation methods that are most enjoyable.

Try not just to recall what you don't like about certain veggies. I've learned it's all about how they are prepared, and often when mixed into something delicious or in a new recipe, you won't mind them one bit. Simply stand in the produce section and look around at your options: perhaps there are some vegetables you have dismissed that deserve another chance, maybe this time prepared an entirely different way and consumed with a smile. Like I tell my kids, "Of course food tastes bad if you frown while you are eating it." Take this seriously; your success at becoming more lean and healthy largely depends on the make up of half your plate!

Excerpt from the *Countdown to Your Best Body Success Journal*, page 47

" I'm very surprised how many veggie-based recipes I liked!"
—TAMMY, 35

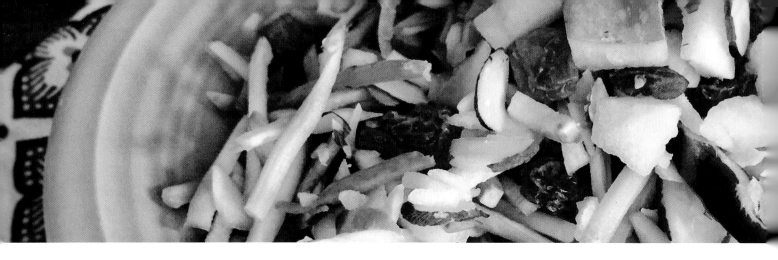

Salad Building 101

Our cookbook offers several different kinds of salad recipes, such as the Refreshing Rainbow Salad pictured. However, we'll often suggest a "green salad" as a side in addition to the recipes offered for the dinner's menu. Or, on evenings when you don't have time to cook, you may just want to toast a pita lightly in the oven while throwing together a quick entree salad with last night's leftover grilled meat on top. When you are building an impromptu salad, consider the following tips.

Be sure that veggies are the star ingredients of your salad. If loaded down with dressing and non-vegetable toppings, salads can be very high in calories.

Don't get bogged down with the same old five ingredients you've always put in your salad. This guide will help you to get creative. Remember, if you allow yourself to get in a rut, eating the same foods all the time, you may tire of healthy eating just before reaching Your Best Body.

Use this quick formula to help you make creative side salads yielding 4 servings:

6 cups greens + 2 cups add-ins + garnishes (amounts listed) + dressing

GREENS:

Red or green leaf lettuce, Boston lettuce, iceberg lettuce, romaine lettuce, baby spinach, baby kale, Swiss chard, bagged salad greens

SALAD ADD-INS:

Shredded cabbage, rainbow slaw, beets, arugula, radicchio, tomatoes, carrots, cucumbers, artichoke hearts, hearts of palm, bell peppers, squash, zucchini, slivered sugar snap peas, celery

GARNISHES OF CHOICE:

- 2–4 tablespoons fresh herbs, such as basil, chives, dill, cilantro, parsley, or oregano

- ¼ to ½ cup sliced or chopped red, yellow or green onion, roasted red peppers, olives, pickled vegetables

- 1-3 tablespoons cheese, nuts, seeds, or dried fruit

  - Feta, goat, blue or parmesan cheese

  - Pecans, walnuts, almonds, pine nuts or peanuts

  - Sesame, sunflower or pumpkin seeds

  - Raisins or other dried fruits (without added sugar, ideally)

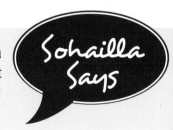

I once worked where there were a bunch of dietitians in one building and we'd have a "salad bar" lunch on Fridays, each bringing a couple of the ingredients above to share. It is an easy and inexpensive way to get have great lunch with friends or colleagues...try it! RDN credentials not required.

SALAD DRESSING:

Use the least amount of salad dressing needed. Start with 1-1½ tablespoons vinaigrette, light vinaigrette, or light creamy dressing per serving.

TO DRESS THE SALAD:

In a large salad bowl, gently toss the greens with the add-ins.

Vinaigrette: Drizzle the dressing over the salad and gently toss until all ingredients are lightly coated with the vinaigrette. Arrange the salad on a serving plate and top with garnishes.

Creamy dressing: Divide the salad among serving plates, drizzle with dressing, top with garnishes and serve (creamy dressings are heavy and weigh down lettuce if tossed).

In a hurry? Just put your salad in a bowl, add dressing and eat. It does not have to be complicated....but Kim admits she likes it to be just a little bit fancy...she even has a favorite salad tossing bowl. My favorite salad is pictured.

For a couple quick examples, see Day 23's **Sweet and Simple Spinach Salad** or Day 43's **4-Ingredient Kale Salad.**

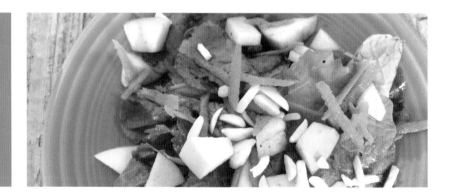

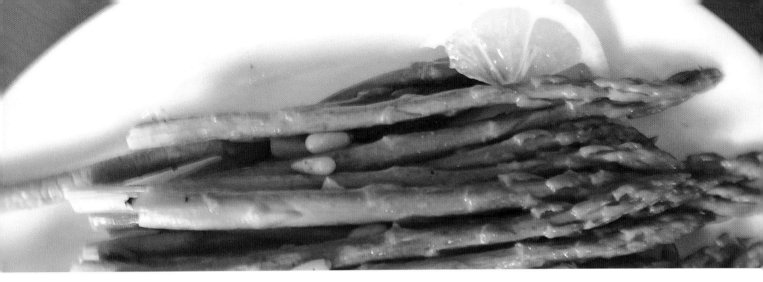

Vegetable Cooking Options

SIMPLE SAUTÉ:

"To sauté" simply means to cook food in hot fat (such as oil or butter). It is best to sauté tender vegetables such as asparagus, bok choy, sugar snap peas, mushrooms, spinach, squash, zucchini and bell peppers.

Cut vegetables into uniform pieces (to promote even cooking).

Heat the pan over medium-high heat, add 1-3 teaspoons oil and spray with cooking spray. Once the oil is hot swirl the pan to coat the bottom, add food in a single layer; stir to promote even cooking and browning.

To sauté less tender vegetables, such as broccoli, Brussels sprouts, cauliflower, potatoes or carrots, first sauté as mentioned above, stirring to coat in oil. Once the vegetables begin to soften, add a little liquid (water, broth or a combination) to the pan. Bring to a slow boil, reduce heat and cover. Cook until the desired degree of doneness is achieved.

STEAMING 3 WAYS:

Steaming is a great choice because it is quick, helps veggies to retain their nutrients, and doesn't require fat.

• Steamer bags are readily available in markets everywhere. Both fresh and frozen vegetables can be steamed in the microwave by simply following the instructions on the bag.

• Steaming vegetables in a microwave-safe bowl is another easy way to steam vegetables if you prefer not to cook in plastic or if you don't buy your vegetables in a bag. Simply place uniformly cut vegetables in a microwave-safe bowl and add 2-4 tablespoons of water; cover the bowl loosely with a paper towel and microwave for 1-3 minutes. At 30-60 second intervals, check for doneness and stir to promote even cooking.

• Stove-top steaming is an equally simple way to steam vegetables. Place a steamer basket filled with uniformly cut vegetables into a sauce pan and add 1-inch of water to the pan. Place the pan over medium-high heat, cover, and cook until the vegetables reach the desired degree of doneness.

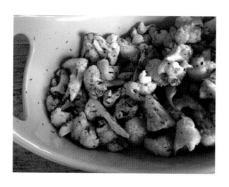

ROASTING:

We both love this method! If you aren't a fan of traditionally prepared vegetables, you really should try roasting them. They taste totally different...and are delicious!

Cut vegetables into uniform pieces and spread them in a single layer on a baking sheet. Add 3-4 teaspoons of oil plus seasonings of choice; toss to coat the vegetables. Cook in a preheated oven at 400-425 degrees. Stir halfway through cooking time. Cook until tender, usually 25-30 minutes.

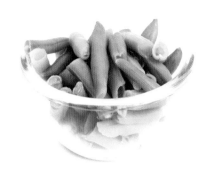 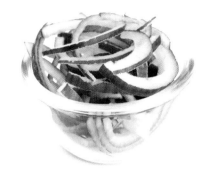 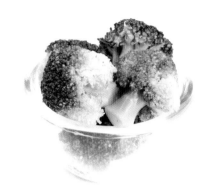

Extras

SEASONING BLENDS

Many of our recipes use seasoning blends in an effort to save you time and reduce the ingredient list length. Over our years as dietitians, we have noticed that people can be discouraged by long ingredient lists, so seasoning blends are a great convenience. Blends are a nice way to add flavor with "one shake." Some blends contain more sodium than others, but we have monitored that in our recipes for you.

Jane's Krazy Mixed-Up Salt® includes salt, dehydrated onion, garlic and dried herbs. Although it is a salt blend, Jane's Krazy Mixed-Up Salt® contains half the sodium of straight salt. If you replace salt in your recipes with this blend you will automatically reduce the sodium to half. If you prefer to use salt instead, simply use half of the amount called for in the recipe and add any other salt-free seasonings you prefer.

Greek seasoning (such as Cavenders®) is another salt blend with a variety of spices and dried herbs used to add a wonderful umami (or savory) flavor to our recipes.

Salt-free blends (such as Mrs. Dash®) come in many varieties that complement a lot of foods. Many times we pair them with salt or another blend containing salt; this adds flavor without increasing the overall salt content in your food.

OILS AND FATS

Most of our recipes call for extra-virgin olive oil or canola oil. These are the two most healthy and versatile oils for your pantry. Canola oil is less expensive, is refined, has a neutral flavor and can withstand higher temperatures. Extra-virgin olive oil is more expensive and less refined therefore it imparts more flavors. It does not withstand high temperatures as well as canola oil. This does not mean they have to be the only two oils you use. Specialty oils are wonderful to experiment with and enjoy. Coconut oil also imparts a nice slightly tropical flavor to cooking and while it is quite trendy, the research does not support use of coconut oil exclusively over other oils. It is important to include a variety of healthy fats in your diet (in moderate amounts), just as it is important to eat a variety of vegetables (in significant amounts).

MILK

When unspecified milk is called for in this cookbook, we are referring to nonfat or 1% milk. Feel free to substitute for a different milk product if desired, keeping in mind that they have different nutritional profiles and varying benefits. Choose your milk based on the nutritional profile that best suits your nutrient needs. For example, use dairy products for cheese and yogurt, use plain soy milk or cow's milk with breakfast for more protein to hold you through the morning, and use almond milk when you need the calories as low as possible and have already met your protein needs for that segment of the day, like when having a treat such as the Coffee and Cream Shake.

Naturally occurring sugar from milk (that does not have sugar added in processing) doesn't count toward your number of grams of daily added sugar, but remember the importance of moderation.

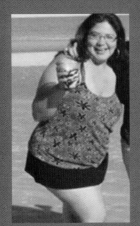
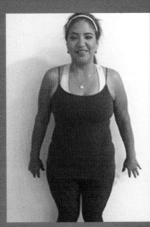
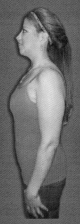

BEFORE   HALFWAY   CURRENT

"I have completed 3 rounds of the Best Body Countdown and lost 65 pounds! I am so happy to have recipes at my fingertips that meet the Countdown criteria for healthy eating! So many favorites!

—ESMERALDA, 46

menu plan

menu plan

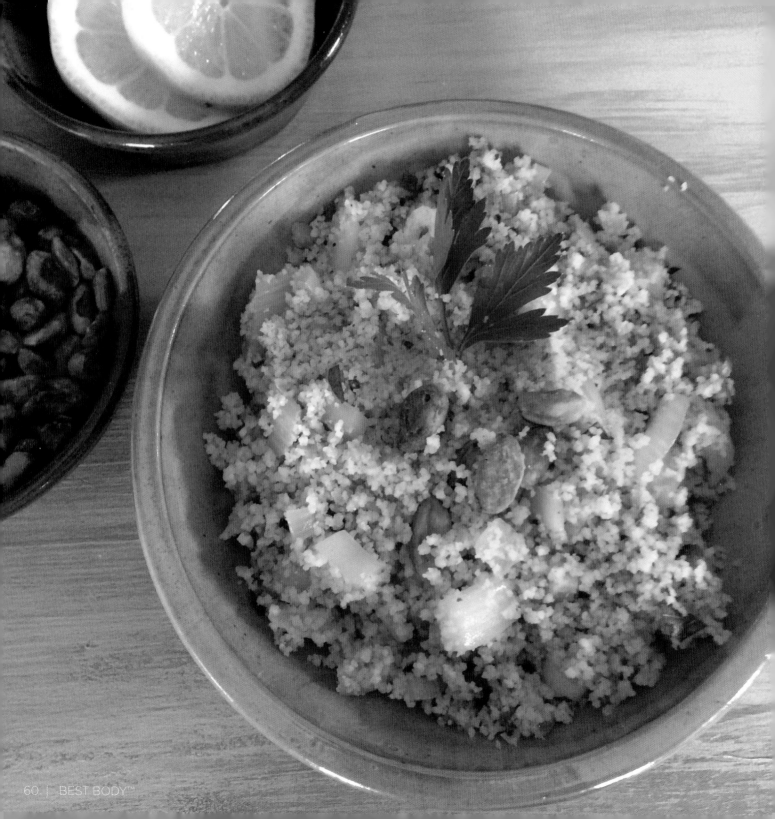

recipes & menu:
week one

<blockquote>
" This recipe is certainly silly. It says to separate two eggs, but it doesn't say how far to separate them."

—GRACIE ALLEN
</blockquote>

menu key:

Lunch Leftovers

Pricey Meal

Quicker-Fix

Slow-Cooker

Club Favorite

Easy Meal

PRE-COUNTDOWN DAY
Garlic Pork Loin
Refreshing Rainbow Salad
Sweet Potato Mirco-Mash

DAY 52 *(typically Tuesday)*
Blackened Cod
Couscous with Pistachios
Suggested side: steamed or sautéed broccoli

Day 51
Easy Asian Stir-Fry

Day 50
Toasted Eggplant Sandwiches
Quinoa Pilaf with Pine Nuts

Day 49
Bruschetta Chicken
Roasted Vegetables with Orzo
Suggested side: green salad

Day 48
Spice-Coated Turkey Burgers
Green Beans with Roasted Red Peppers

Day 47
Steak with Mushroom Gravy and Broccoli
Suggested side: green salad

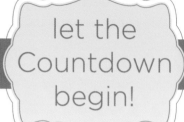

let the Countdown begin!

garlic pork loin

Hands-on time: 15-20 minutes | Total time: 1 hour and 20 minutes
(plus marinating time, 2 hours to overnight)

Club Favorite

Lunch Leftovers

This is a simple way to cook a whole pork loin — enough to eat now and plenty for later. The Easy Asian Stir-Fry recipe on Day 51 turns leftover pork into a delicious "planned over" meal, as does next week's Cocoa-Spiced Pork.

1 3-pound pork loin, trimmed of fat

3–5 large garlic cloves, minced

2 teaspoons Jane's Krazy Mixed-Up Salt

Cracked black pepper, to taste

GROCERY LIST:
Garlic cloves (3–5)

Boneless pork loin (approximately 3 pounds)

Jane's Krazy Mixed-Up Salt

Cracked black pepper

1. Using a knife, make tiny slits all over the meat on both sides and insert minced garlic pieces, pushing them into the meat.
2. Rub seasoning and pepper over both sides of the loin.
3. Refrigerate for at least 2 hours or overnight.
4. When ready to cook, preheat the broiler and place pork on a roasting pan (or a 9x13-inch pan) covered with foil.
5. Broil for 10 minutes on each side or until golden.
6. Turn the oven down to 400°F. Continue roasting for 30–40 minutes or until the internal temperature of the pork registers 145°F on a meat thermometer.
7. Remove the pork from the oven and turn it over, then tent (cover loosely) with foil. Let the meat rest for 5 minutes (the meat will continue to cook with residual heat, and the juices will redistribute, making it more juicy).
8. Slice the loin thinly and enjoy! Refrigerate or freeze leftovers for use later in recipes or as sandwich.

Yield: 10 servings
(serving size: 3 ounces)
Use extras for sandwiches or freeze

Nutrient Breakdown:
Calories 152

Fat 5g
(2g saturated fat)

Cholesterol 70mg

Sodium 300mg

Carbohydrate 0g

Fiber 0g

Protein 24g

Plate Plan choices:
3 lean meats
(3 ounces)

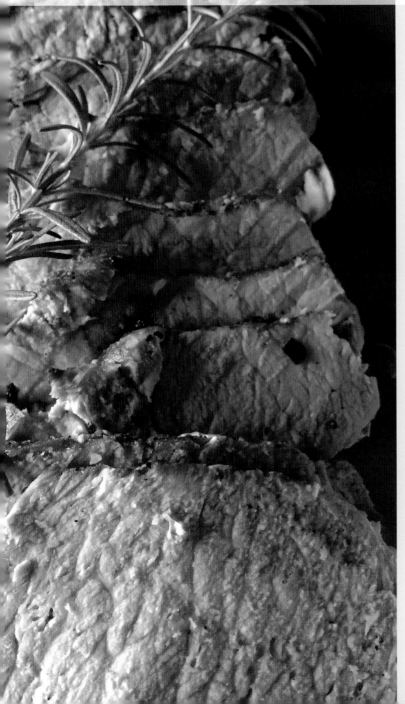

"Lemons, garlic and herbs, oh my!"

LEMONS: As you read through the recipes, you will notice many are served with lemons and occasionally limes. The juice (acid) heightens other flavors and adds brightness to food. In fact, lemons enhance the flavor of salt, so when you're tempted to add more salt, try a little squeeze of lemon instead. We recommend keeping lemons and limes as a pantry staple and keeping some lemon juice to use when fresh lemons are not handy (even Kim admits to using the little plastic fruit when time is tight).

GARLIC: A head or bulb of garlic has sections when you peel it; each section is a clove of garlic. One medium clove of garlic equals about 1 teaspoon minced garlic and about ¼ teaspoon garlic powder. Though fresh garlic is our favorite, you can find jarred minced garlic or garlic paste in the produce section or freezer section of the store for a suitable, quicker option.

HERBS: In our recipes, both fresh and dried herbs are used. If fresh herbs are called for, the recipe will say "fresh," otherwise it is a dried herb. Please feel free to substitute fresh for dry herbs or vice versa. The general guideline is to use one-third the amount of dry herbs when substituting for fresh. When replacing dry with fresh herbs, use three times the amount of fresh.

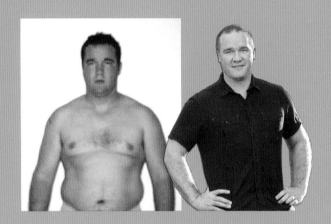

"My wife, who does most of the cooking, was able to stay motivated during the Best Body Countdown because she did not have to cook two separate meals for our family. Being able to enjoy foods together, that everyone liked, made meal time seem special. The Refreshing Rainbow Salad is a favorite!"

—JASON, 38

*To toast nuts, place a dry, nonstick skillet over medium heat and add nuts. Toast the nuts for 2–4 minutes, stirring or shaking the pan frequently to avoid burning. As they become fragrant and begin to change color, remove them from the heat. You can even toast a bunch at one time and store them in the refrigerator for future use!

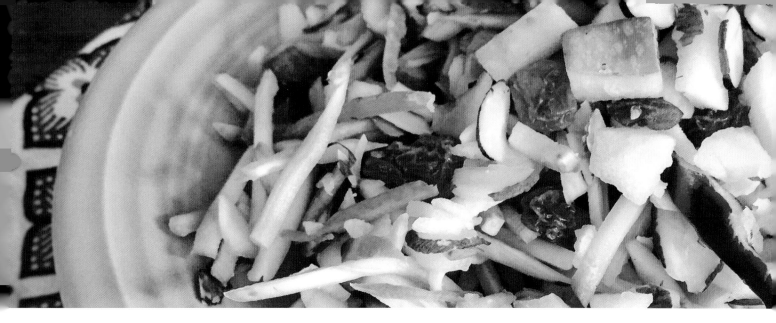

refreshing rainbow salad

Total time: 15 minutes

Lunch Leftovers

The sweet, tart flavor combined with the crunchy texture of this simple slaw appeals to those who may not enjoy a typical leafy green salad.

½ 12-ounce bag of rainbow slaw (also called California slaw or broccoli slaw)

1 Granny Smith apple, washed, cored and cut in quarters (do not remove peel)

3–4 teaspoons lemon juice

½ cup slivered almonds, toasted* (toasting is optional, but optimal)

½ cup golden raisins

GROCERY LIST:
12-ounce bag of rainbow slaw (also called California Slaw or broccoli slaw)

Granny smith apple (1)

Lemon or lemon juice

Slivered almonds (½ cup)

Golden raisins (½ cup)

1. Briefly pulse the apple (6 pulses) in a food processor or blender. Add the slaw and briefly pulse (2 pulses, just enough to make sure the big pieces are bite-sized). Note: The other half of the bag of slaw will be used on Day 51 in the Easy Asian Stir-Fry.

2. Transfer slaw mix to a large bowl. Add the lemon juice, almonds, and raisins.

3. Toss and serve promptly.

Yield: 6 servings
(serving size: generous ½ cup)

Nutrient Breakdown:
Calories 127

Fat 5g

Carbohydrate 19g

Fiber 7g

Sodium 12mg

Protein 3g

(This recipe has 4g of sugar, all from fruit, so none of it is considered added sugar.)

Plate Plan choices:
1 fruit, 1 vegetable, 1 fat

sweet potato micro-mash

This is the easiest way to make sweet potatoes: simply microwave and mash. If you can find them fresh at the farmer's market, they will be even more delightful! This would be a great time to cook an extra potato for use in the Sweet Potato Oat Pancakes recipe.

2 sweet potatoes, scrubbed clean, with peel

GROCERY LIST:
Sweet potatoes (2)

Seasoning(s) of choice (see suggestions)

1. Pierce the sweet potato skin 5–6 times with a fork or knife.

2. Place on a microwave-safe plate and microwave for 5–8 minutes, rotating halfway through.

3. The sweet potato is done when the thin skin puffs to a crisp finish; the inside will be tender and moist. Remove the flesh from the peel while holding the potato with an oven mitt to avoid burns. Mash and season as desired.

Yield: 4 servings
(*serving size: ½ cup*)

Nutrient Breakdown:
Calories 60

Sodium 35mg

Carbohydrate 13g

Fiber 2g

Protein 1g

Plate Plan choices:
1 starch

seasoning suggestions:

1 teaspoon healthy fat
+ tiny pinch of salt

allspice + cinnamon + ginger

cinnamon + cilantro + lime

rosemary + pumpkin seeds

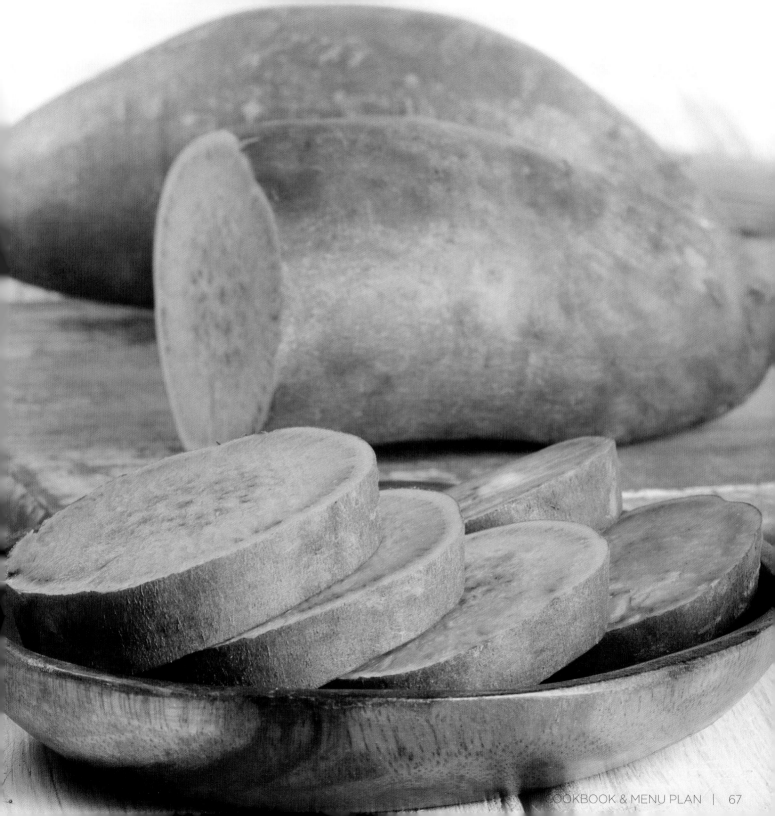

PREPARING FISH: FRESH AND FROZEN

Frozen fish is a wonderful product; it is usually flash-frozen soon after it is caught, so it maintains a high level of freshness. Of course, fresh (never frozen) fish is ideal, but unless you live on the coast, it can be difficult to come by. In fact, most of the fish at the grocer's fish counter comes in frozen, and they thaw it out to display and sell.

To get the freshest fish from the fish counter, ask some basic questions. Find out when the fish came in, ask if it has been frozen, and if so, how long it has been thawed. Use your senses to evaluate: does it look firm and fresh? Does it smell overly fishy? Fish should look firm and smell fresh (a bit like the ocean).

While thawing, or in preparation to cook the fish, giving it a soak in milk will help to freshen it and reduce any fishy odor.

Thaw fish by removing the packaging and placing the fish in a shallow dish or plastic zip-top bag. Add about 1 cup of milk (per 4 fillets) to the fish, seal, and thaw overnight in the refrigerator.

If using fresh fish, place it in a shallow dish or pie plate and pour milk over the fish, allowing it to soak while you gather the remaining ingredients. When you're ready to cook, remove the fish from the milk, pat dry with towels, and cook as directed.

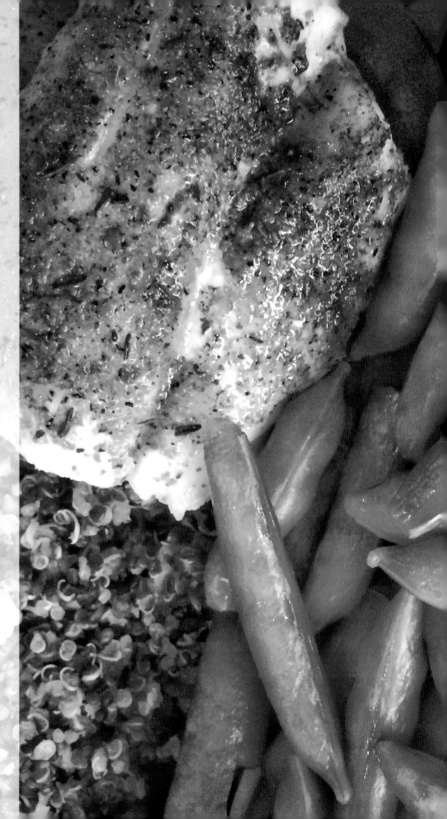

DAY 52

Easy Meal

blackened cod

Total time: 20 minutes
(allow fish to thaw overnight in the refrigerator)

Simple can be delicious! This recipe makes that statement loud and clear. The mild taste of cod is perfectly accentuated by the blackened seasoning and lime juice. Cooking fish doesn't have to be intimidating. In this recipe, we present fabulously simple baked or sautéed options that will have you on your way to cooking flavorful fish any day of the week.

suggested side: steamed or sautéed broccoli

4 4–5-ounce frozen or fresh cod fillets (soak or thaw in milk, if desired; see feature)

Canola oil cooking spray

2 tablespoons lime juice plus lime wedges for serving

4 teaspoons blackened redfish seasoning (such as Chef Paul Prudhomme's Magic Seasoning)

GROCERY LIST:
Lime or lime juice (lime wedges are optional)

Frozen cod fillets (4)

Milk (optional)

Chef Paul Prudhomme's Blackened Redfish seasoning

Canola oil cooking spray

Broccoli (suggested side)

1. Preheat the oven to 350°F. Spray a 9x13-inch baking pan with cooking spray. (See note if you prefer to sauté the fish.)

2. Pat fish dry with paper towels, and place in the prepared baking dish. Drizzle the lime juice over the fish and sprinkle seasoning on both sides. Bake for 12–14 minutes or until done (fish is done when it is just opaque throughout).

Yield: 4 servings
(serving size 1 fillet)

Nutrient Breakdown:
Calories 100

Fat 1g (140mg omega-3 fatty acids)

Cholesterol 41mg

Sodium 230mg

Carbohydrate 1g

Protein 21g

Plate Plan choices:
3 very lean meats

If you prefer to sauté, pat the fish dry with paper towels and sprinkle both sides with seasoning. Coat a nonstick skillet with cooking spray and add one teaspoon oil. (The cooking spray allows for less use of oil, and it helps the oil spread more evenly across the pan.)

Place over medium heat. Once hot, swirl the oil to coat the pan and add the cod. Cook for 3–4 minutes, flip and cook until done (2– 4 minutes). Serve with lime juice or wedges.

couscous with pistachios

Total time: 20 minutes

Lunch Leftovers

This is a delightfully fluffy side dish with a great flavor.

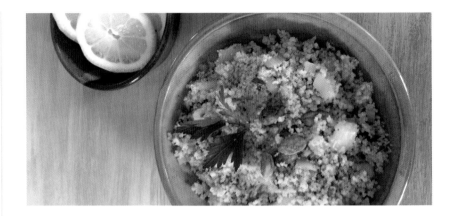

Canola oil cooking spray

1 teaspoon extra-virgin olive oil

1 small onion, diced (about 1 cup)

2 ribs celery, diced

1½ cups reduced-sodium chicken broth

1 cup whole-wheat couscous

1 teaspoon Jane's Krazy Mixed-Up Salt

½ cup pistachios, chopped

¼ cup chopped parsley

Lime wedges to serve

GROCERY LIST:
Parsley
Onion (1 small)
Celery (2 stalks)
Whole-wheat couscous (1 cup)
Fresh lime (wedges for serving)
Pistachios (½ cup)
Reduced-sodium chicken broth
Extra-virgin olive oil
Jane's Krazy Mixed-Up Salt
Canola oil cooking spray

1. Coat the bottom of a large nonstick skillet with cooking spray, add oil, and place over medium heat. Once hot, add the onion and celery. Cook until soft (about 2 minutes), stirring occasionally.

2. Add broth to the skillet and bring to a boil. Stir in couscous and salt, cover, and remove from heat. Let stand 5 minutes.

3. Once the couscous is done, mix in the pistachios and parsley and fluff with a fork. Serve with lime. (If you decide to use this recipe for leftovers, wait to add the pistachios until it's time to serve).

Yield: 8 servings
(serving size: ½ cup)

Nutrient Breakdown:
Calories 130

Fat 4.5g (0g saturated fat, 2g monounsaturated fat)

Sodium 180mg

Carbohydrate 21g

Fiber 4g

Protein 5g

Plate Plan choices:
1 starch, ½ vegetable, 1 fat

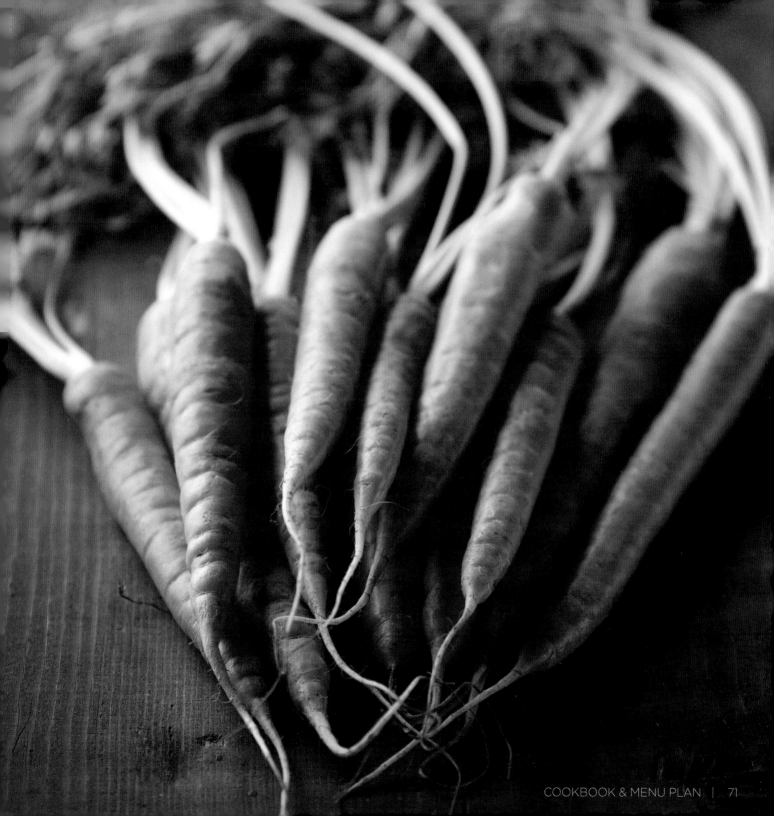

Easy Meal

easy asian stir-fry

Total time: 20 minutes

Lunch Leftovers

Club Favorite

Everyone loves this simple stir-fry. Next time, try it with chicken for a twist. Either way, it's a recipe you will want to keep on hand. Though it's a veggie-loaded entrée, none of the vegetables has an overpowering flavor. This is Sohailla's kids' favorite!

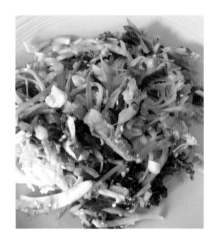

You may be tempted to use whatever oil you have on hand, but we don't suggest skimping here. Sesame oil, found on the Asian food aisle at the grocery store, is a fabulous flavor enhancer that we use in a few recipes during the Countdown. A little goes a long way! *(Tip: keep it in your refrigerator once opened.)*

1 7-ounce package brown rice noodles

1 tablespoon canola oil

½ 12-ounce bag of rainbow slaw (left over from making the Refreshing Rainbow Salad)

2 ounces kale cut into bite-sized pieces (3 cups, packed)

1 bag Asian-blend chopped salad (such as Dole), use only veggies, not the condiments

⅓ cup thinly sliced green onions

2 cups unsalted chicken broth, divided

1½ tablespoons cornstarch

4 tablespoons reduced-sodium soy sauce

1 teaspoon sesame oil

1½ teaspoon fresh grated ginger (or in the tube)

2 cloves garlic, minced

1½ pounds precooked pork loin, *in bite-size strips

3 tablespoons toasted sesame seeds

GROCERY LIST:
Rainbow slaw mix (if you don't have ½ bag remaining from Pre-Countdown Day)

Kale (2 ounces)

Asian-blend chopped salad (1 bag)

Green onions

Fresh ginger or ginger in the tube

Garlic cloves (2)

Pork loin (1½ pounds if you do not have leftovers)

Brown rice noodles (7-ounce package)

Sesame seeds (3 tablespoons)

Unsalted chicken broth

Reduced-sodium soy sauce

Cornstarch

Sesame oil

Canola oil

Yield: 6 servings

(serving size: 2 cups pork mixture and ¾ cup noodles)

Nutrient Breakdown:

Calories 450

Fat 16g (3.5g saturated fat)

Cholesterol 90mg

Sodium 670mg

Carbohydrate 38g

Fiber 6g

Protein 34g

Plate Plan choices:

2 starches, 2 vegetables, 4 very lean meats, 1 fat

1. Cook the noodles according to package directions.

2. Add oil to a large nonstick skillet and place over medium heat. Once the oil is hot, swirl to coat the pan. Add the rainbow slaw, kale, chopped salad, and onions and stir to combine. If the pan is a little dry, add up to ¼ cup of chicken broth to facilitate cooking. Cook for 4 minutes, cover with a lid and cook 2 more minutes.

3. Next, prepare the coating sauce. In a medium bowl, stir together the cornstarch and ¼ cup chicken broth until smooth. Add the remaining chicken broth, soy sauce, sesame oil, ginger and garlic. Stir to combine.

4. Once the vegetables are cooked, add the pork, sesame seeds, and coating sauce to the pan (if the sauce sits too long, it may be necessary to re-mix, as the cornstarch will settle at the bottom). Bring the mixture to a boil for a minimum of one minute and allow the sauce to thicken. Cook until the pork is heated through (about 3 minutes). Serve over brown rice noodles.

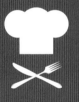

*If using fresh uncooked pork, cut the pork into bite-size strips (about ¼-inch wide). Spray a large nonstick skillet with cooking spray, add ½ tablespoon canola oil and place over medium-high heat. When the oil is hot, add the pork to the pan and sauté for 3–4 minutes or until done. With a slotted spoon or tongs, transfer the pork to a plate and tent with aluminum foil to keep warm. Proceed with the recipe as directed.

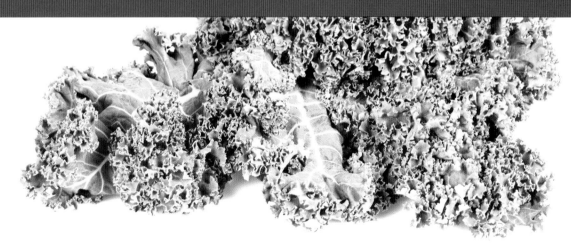

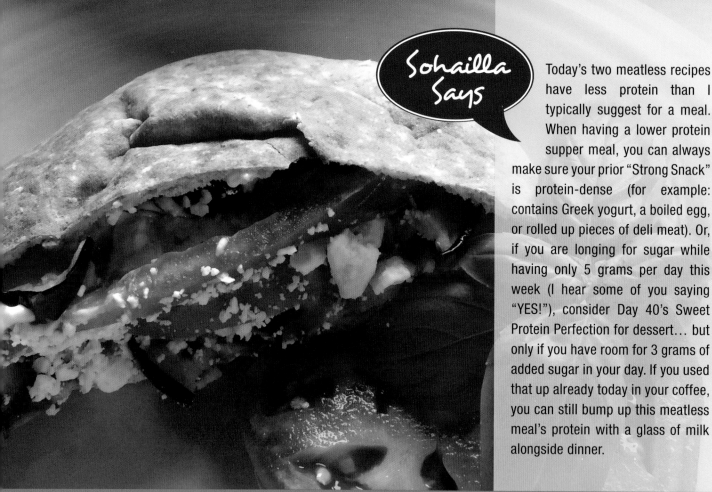

DAY 50

toasted eggplant sandwiches

Total time: 30 minutes

Club Favorite

These are a Best Body Club favorite you'll be making for years to come! They often score a 10 out of 10 on our taste tests. Even if you don't think you like eggplant, after trying this, you just might. Give it a try!

1 small eggplant, peeled and cut into ¼-inch slices (about 16 slices)

Canola oil cooking spray

½ cup canola mayonnaise (our preference, similar to light mayonnaise)

3 cloves of garlic, minced

¼ cup chopped fresh basil

2 whole-wheat pita rounds, cut into 4 halves

2 tomatoes, thinly sliced

½ cup crumbled feta cheese (2 ounces)

GROCERY LIST:
Eggplant (1 pound)

Tomatoes (2)

Garlic cloves (3)

Fresh basil

Whole-wheat pita rounds (2)

Feta cheese (½ cup crumbled)

Canola mayonnaise

Canola oil cooking spray

Salad fixings (suggested side)

1. Preheat oven to 400°F. Lightly spray eggplant slices with cooking spray and put them in a single layer on a foil-lined baking sheet. Place the eggplant in the oven about 6 inches from the heat source. Cook for 10 minutes on each side.

2. In a small bowl, stir together the mayonnaise, garlic and basil.

3. While the eggplant cooks, lightly toast the pita in the oven, about 2 minutes.

4. To build the pita sandwich, place two slices of eggplant in the pita pocket, laying them against one side of the pita. Spread 1–2 tablespoons of mayonnaise mixture on the eggplant slices. Top the mayonnaise mixture with two slices tomato, then top with two more slices of eggplant. Sprinkle feta cheese into the pita.

Yield: 4 servings
(serving size: 1 sandwich made from half of a pita round)

Nutrient Breakdown:
Calories 250

Fat 12g (1.5g saturated fat)

Carbohydrate 27g

Sodium 580mg

Fiber 7g

Protein 7g

Plate Plan choices:
1 starch, 2 vegetables, equivalent to ½ serving of medium-fat meat, 2 fats

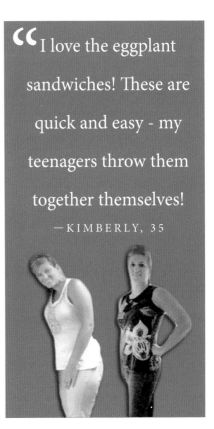

" I love the eggplant sandwiches! These are quick and easy - my teenagers throw them together themselves!
— KIMBERLY, 35

Sohailla Says

This was adapted from a recipe a friend of mine gave me about 10 years ago and has been one of our family favorites ever since. My kids like it best when I add thin turkey pepperoni slices to their loaded pita rounds as well. To dress this up on occasion, use crusty French bread slices in the place of pita rounds. Yum!

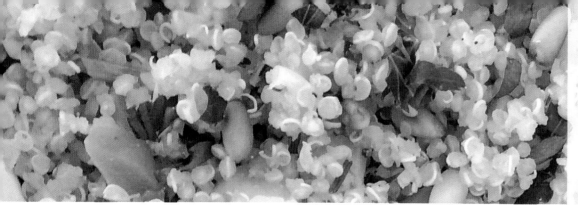

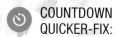

COUNTDOWN QUICKER-FIX:
Use precooked or microwavable quinoa. Follow directions as below, following steps 1, 2, and 4.

quinoa pilaf with pine nuts

Total time: 25 minutes

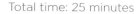

Quicker-Fix

Lunch Leftovers

Want something just a little different than standard rice? Give quinoa a try! It's a seed that cooks up much like a grain—in about 20 minutes. It can be substituted for rice in many recipes.

Canola oil cooking spray

1 teaspoon extra-virgin olive oil

1 cup frozen chopped mirepoix mix of onion, celery, and carrot (if using fresh vegetables, use ½ cup chopped onion, 1 celery stalk and 1 carrot, chopped)

2 garlic cloves, minced

½ cup quinoa, rinsed and drained

1 cup reduced-sodium broth

¼ cup water

½ teaspoon Jane's Krazy Mixed-Up Salt

¼ cup toasted pine nuts

2 tablespoons chopped parsley (optional garnish)

1. Spray a large pot or Dutch oven with cooking spray, add oil and place over medium heat.
2. Once the oil is hot, add the mirepoix and garlic to the pan and cook for 2–3 minutes, or until tender.
3. Stir in quinoa, broth, water and salt. Bring to a boil. Reduce heat and simmer for 20 minutes until the water is absorbed.
4. Toss with pine nuts and parsley just before serving.

Yield: 4 servings
(serving size: ½ cup)

Nutrient Breakdown:
Calories 170

Fat 6g (0g saturated fat)

Cholesterol 0mg

Sodium 220mg

Carbohydrate 23g

Fiber 10g

Protein 5g

Plate Plan choices:
1 starch

GROCERY LIST:
Garlic cloves (2)

Parsley (optional)

Quinoa (½ cup)

Pine nuts (¼ cup)

Reduced-sodium vegetable or chicken broth

Frozen chopped mirepoix mix or onion, celery, carrot

Extra-virgin olive oil

Canola oil cooking spray

Jane's Krazy Mixed-Up Salt

DAY 49

While Bruschetta Chicken is cooking, prepare the Roasted Vegetables with Orzo recipe. Both cook in a 400°F oven, but the chicken takes twice as long to cook, so you have approximately 15 minutes to prep your vegetables before they need to go in.

bruschetta chicken

Lunch Leftovers

Club Favorite

This recipe can be assembled quickly and is super flavorful. Panko breadcrumbs are available with different seasonings: feel free to choose any flavor. As an alternative to panko, make your own breadcrumbs using whole-grain or gluten-free bread. Simply toast the bread and pulse in a food processor.

1 14.5-ounce can no-salt-added diced tomatoes, undrained

1½ cups Italian flavored panko breadcrumbs (½ of an 8-ounce package)

2 cloves garlic, minced

1½ pounds boneless, skinless chicken breasts (cut into bitesized pieces)

1 cup shredded part-skim mozzarella cheese

GROCERY LIST:
Garlic cloves (2)

Boneless, skinless chicken breasts (1½ pounds)

Italian flavored panko bread crumbs (1½ cups)

No-salt-added diced tomatoes (14.5-ounce can)

Part-skim mozzarella cheese (1 cup)

Asparagus (suggested side)

1. Preheat oven to 400°F.

2. Pour tomatoes and their juice into a medium bowl.

3. Add the panko and garlic to the tomatoes and mix until the panko is just moist. If you need more liquid, add hot water 1 tablespoon at a time.

4. Place the chicken in a 9x13-inch baking dish and evenly distribute the cheese over the chicken. Top with the breadcrumb mixture and bake for 30 minutes.

Hands-on time: 15 minutes
Total time: 45 minutes

Yield: 6 servings
(serving size: about 1¼ cups)

Nutrient Breakdown: Calories 260

Fat 7g (3g saturated fat)

Cholesterol 85mg

Sodium 400mg

Carbohydrate 18g

Fiber 2g

Protein 31g

Plate Plan choices:
1 starch, 1 vegetable, 4 lean meats

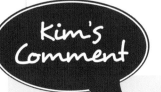
Kim's Comment

Originally, we tried this with stuffing mix, but to our dismay, all the stuffing mixes available contained partially hydrogenated oil (trans fat). However, seasoned panko breadcrumbs make a delightful substitution and have a much cleaner ingredient list. Remember, using homemade breadcrumbs from toasted whole-grain bread works, too!

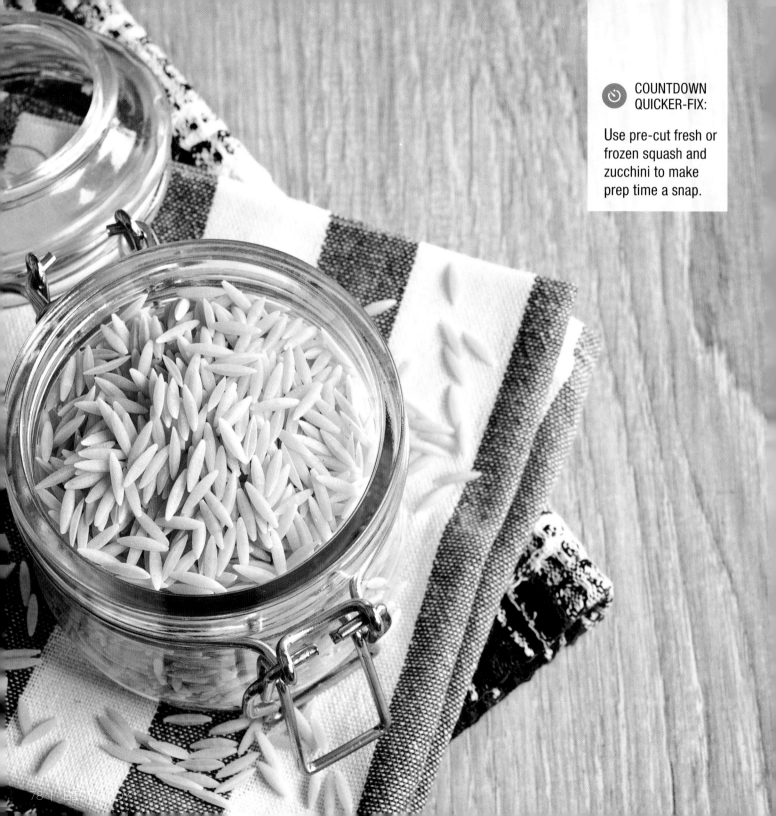

*You can easily mix these vegetables with any leftover or microwaveable whole grain, such as barley, rice, or couscous.

roasted vegetables with orzo

Total time: 25 minutes

Quicker-Fix

Lunch Leftovers

This recipe incorporates several flavor and convenience techniques. Roasting vegetables is a great flavor enhancer, while roasted red peppers from the jar provide an effortless punch of flavor and color. This recipe makes plenty, so you can cook once and eat twice (or more). Pair this with cooked chicken for a great "Lunch Leftover."

Canola oil cooking spray

2 medium zucchini, chopped (about 3 cups)

2 medium yellow squash, chopped (about 2½ cups)

1 small onion, chopped (about 1 cup)

1 large garlic clove, minced

2 teaspoons Jane's Krazy Mixed-Up Salt

1 teaspoon dried thyme

2 teaspoons extra-virgin olive oil

1 cup reduced-sodium chicken broth

2 cups water

2 cups whole-wheat orzo or whole grain of choice*

⅓ cup chopped roasted red pepper (from jar)

Parsley (optional garnish)

1. Preheat the oven to 400°F. Line a large baking sheet with aluminum foil and spray with cooking spray.

2. In a large bowl combine the zucchini, yellow squash, onion and garlic with seasoning salt, thyme and oil. Toss to coat in oil. Spread the vegetables out in a single layer on the prepared baking sheet. Roast for 15–18 minutes, stirring halfway through cooking time.

3. While the vegetables roast, bring the broth and water to a boil. Reduce the heat and add orzo, stirring frequently, adding more water if needed. Cook until done (about 9 minutes) and drain any remaining liquid off of the orzo.

4. Combine the red pepper, roasted vegetables and orzo. Serve with parsley, if desired.

Yield: 8 servings
(serving size: 1 cup)

Nutrient Breakdown:
Calories 100

Fat 1.5g
(0g saturated fat)

Cholesterol 0mg

Sodium 380mg

Carbohydrate 8g

Fiber 3g

Protein 4g

Plate Plan choices:
1 starch,
1 vegetable

GROCERY LIST:
Zucchini (2 medium)

Yellow squash (2 medium)

Onion (1 small)

Garlic clove (1)

Parsley (optional)

Whole-wheat orzo (2 cups)

Roasted red pepper from jar (⅓ cup)

Reduced-sodium chicken broth

Jane's Krazy Mixed-Up Salt

Dried thyme

Extra-virgin olive oil

Canola cooking spray

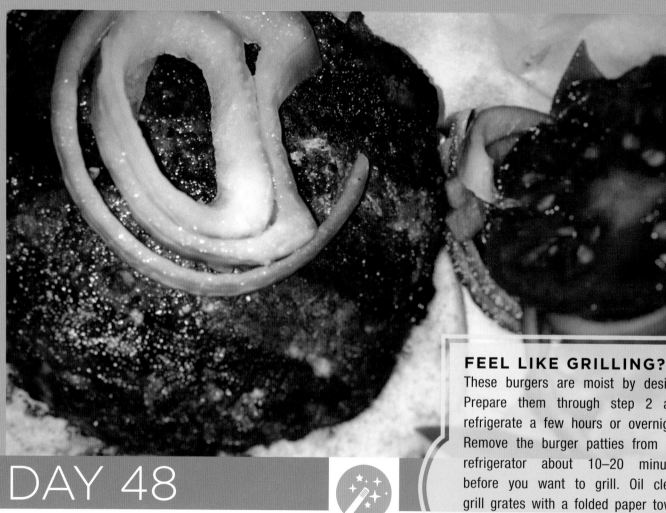

DAY 48

Easy Meal

spice-coated turkey burgers

These are Kim's favorite turkey burgers!

Total time: 20 minutes

FEEL LIKE GRILLING?
These burgers are moist by design. Prepare them through step 2 and refrigerate a few hours or overnight. Remove the burger patties from the refrigerator about 10–20 minutes before you want to grill. Oil clean grill grates with a folded paper towel soaked in canola oil. Preheat the grill to medium and place the burgers on the grill. Keeping the grill lid closed, cook for 5–6 minutes per side, or until the internal temperature registers 165°F degrees on a meat thermometer.

If you are wondering if you can just go with regular paprika, the answer is, sure!
(But Kim says you'd be missing out.)

Burgers:

1 pound ground turkey breast

1 tablespoon canola mayonnaise

1½ teaspoon extra-virgin olive oil, divided

¼ cup finely chopped red onion

Canola oil cooking spray

4 whole-wheat buns or sandwich thins

4 lettuce leaves

4 thin tomato slices

Red onion slices (optional, but delicious)

Spice rub:

3 teaspoons Jane's Krazy Mixed-Up Salt

1 teaspoon chili powder

1 teaspoon smoked paprika

1. In a large bowl, combine the ground turkey with mayonnaise, ½ teaspoon oil, and onion. Mix, taking care not to overmix. Divide the turkey into 4 equal burger patties and pat as thin as possible (but not so thin that they start to fall apart)—this facilitates cooking more quickly to avoid dry burgers.

2. In a small bowl, mix the spices for the rub and transfer them to a plate. Dredge each burger through the rub to coat both sides in spice.

3. Place a nonstick skillet coated with cooking spray over medium to medium low heat and add remaining oil. Once oil is hot, add the burger patties.

4. Cook for 3 minutes on one side and flip. Cook another 3 minutes and then add 2 tablespoons of water to the pan, cover with the lid, and cook for another 2 minutes or until done. Burgers are done when the internal temperature registers 165°F on a meat thermometer. Serve on a bun or sandwich thins with lettuce, tomatoes, and toppings of choice.

Yield: 4 servings
(serving size: 1 burger with bun)

Nutrient Breakdown:
Calories 320

Fat 14g
(2.5g saturated fat, 3g monounsaturated fat)

Cholesterol 45mg

Sodium 710mg

Carbohydrate 24g

Fiber 4g

Protein 24g

Plate Plan choices:
1½ starches, 3 lean meats, 1 fat

GROCERY LIST:

Lettuce

Tomato (1)

Red onion (½ small onion)

Ground turkey breast (1 pound)

Whole-wheat buns (4)

Canola mayonnaise

Jane's Krazy Mixed-Up Salt

Chili powder

Smoked paprika

Extra-virgin olive oil

Canola oil cooking spray

TOPPING SUGGESTIONS

Light cheese: 1 slice – 70 calories, 4.5g fat (3g saturated fat), 170mg sodium, 8g protein

Ketchup: 1 tablespoon – 15 calories, 0g fat, 90mg sodium, 4g carbohydrate

Mayonnaise: 1 tablespoon – 100 calories, 11g fat (1.5g saturated fat), 75mg sodium

Light mayonnaise: 1 tablespoon – 50 calories, 5g fat (1g saturated fat), 105mg sodium

Canola Mayonnaise: 1 tablespoon – 40 calories, 4g fat (0g saturated fat), 115mg sodium

Avocado: 1/5th – 50 calories, 4.5g fat (0.5g saturated fat), 2g fiber

Mustard: 1 teaspoon – 0 calories, 0g fat, 60mg sodium

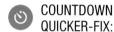

COUNTDOWN QUICKER-FIX:

Simply steam the green beans and toss with oil, pepper and seasoning salt.

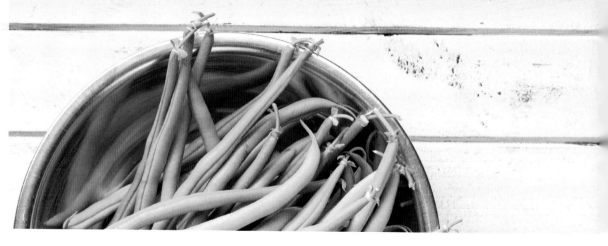

green beans with roasted red peppers

Quicker-Fix

The contrast of color and flavor in this vegetable combination truly makes this dish great for family and guests alike!

Total time: 7 minutes

1 12-ounce microwavable package of fresh green beans

½ tablespoon extra-virgin olive oil

¼ cup chopped roasted red pepper (from jar)

2 cloves garlic, minced

½ teaspoon Jane's Krazy Mixed-Up Salt

GROCERY LIST:
Fresh green beans (12-ounce bag)

Garlic cloves (2)

Roasted red peppers, jarred

Extra-virgin olive oil

Jane's Krazy Mixed-Up Salt

1. Steam green beans (either as directed on the package or in a microwave-safe bowl). To steam green beans in a bowl, place trimmed green beans in a microwave-safe bowl with ¼ cup water and cover with a damp paper towel. Microwave for 2–4 minutes (depending on how tender you like your green beans).

2. Add the oil to a large nonstick skillet and place over medium-high heat. Once the oil is hot, add the roasted red peppers and garlic and cook for 30 seconds. Add the drained green beans and salt. Stir to combine.

Yield: 4 servings
(serving size: about 1 cup)

Nutrient Breakdown:
Calories 60

Fat 2g

Cholesterol 0mg

Sodium 230mg

Carbohydrate 8g

Fiber 3g

Protein 2g

Plate Plan choices:
2 vegetables

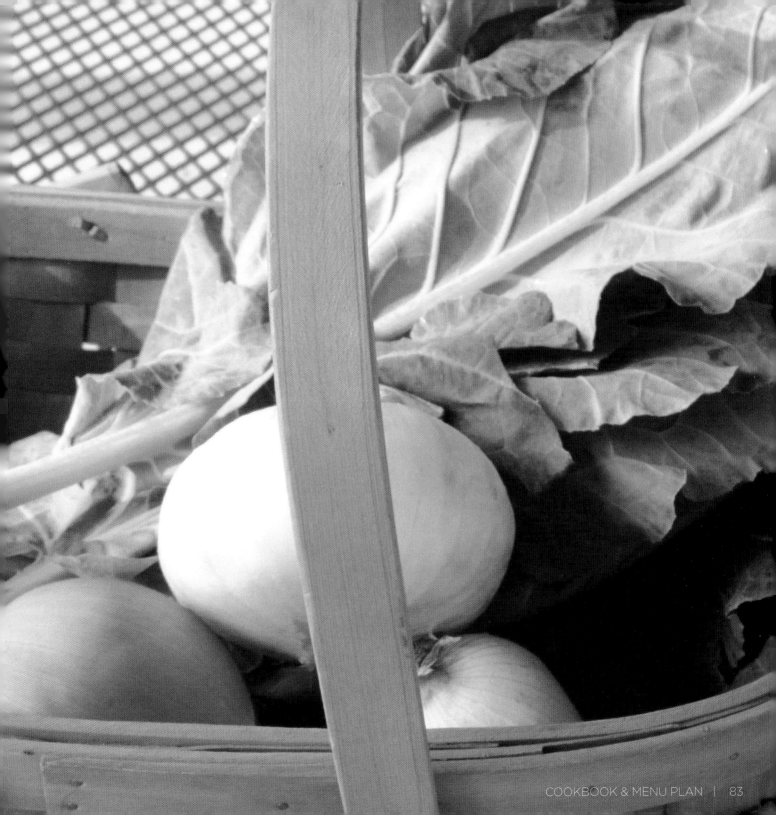

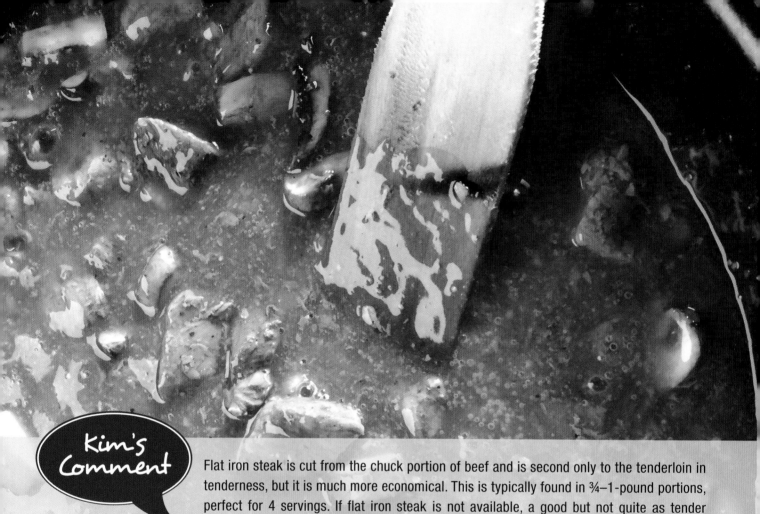

Flat iron steak is cut from the chuck portion of beef and is second only to the tenderloin in tenderness, but it is much more economical. This is typically found in ¾–1-pound portions, perfect for 4 servings. If flat iron steak is not available, a good but not quite as tender substitute is top sirloin steak fillets.

DAY 47

steak with mushroom gravy and broccoli

Pricey Meal

Considered comfort food by many, steak and gravy is delicious but not always healthy. This is a healthful meal: a quarter plate of whole grains, lots of vegetables, and just enough steak to enjoy.

suggested side: green salad

Total time: 30 minutes

¾–1 pound flat iron steak, cut into bite-sized pieces (about ¾ inch)

1 teaspoon salt-free seasoning (such as Original Mrs. Dash)

½ teaspoon salt

Canola oil cooking spray

½ tablespoon canola oil

6 cups chopped broccoli (cut into large pieces)

⅓ cup finely diced onions

1 cup sliced mushrooms

1¾ cup reduced-sodium beef broth, divided

2 tablespoons cornstarch

2 cups cooked brown rice (or precooked)

2 tablespoons chopped fresh parsley (optional garnish)

GROCERY LIST:
Broccoli (6 cups)

Onion

Mushrooms

Parsley (optional)

Flat iron steak (¾–1 pound)

Brown rice (2 cups precooked or microwavable)

Reduced-sodium beef broth

Cornstarch

Original Mrs. Dash

Salt

Canola oil

Canola oil cooking spray

Salad fixings (suggested side)

1. Place the steak and seasoning into a plastic zip-top bag and squish the meat around in the bag to coat thoroughly with seasonings.

2. Coat a large nonstick skillet with cooking spray, add canola oil, and place over medium-high heat. Once the oil is hot, swirl to coat the pan and add the steak in a single layer (divide into 2 batches for cooking if necessary). The steak should sizzle when added to the pan. Cook the meat undisturbed for 45 seconds. Stir the meat and allow it to sear on a second side for 45 seconds, stir again and cook until the meat is done (1–2 minutes more). Remove the meat to a plate and tent with aluminum foil to keep warm. If cooking in batches, repeat the procedure with second batch of meat.

3. Place a steamer basket in a large saucepan. Add broccoli to the basket and fill the pan with 1 inch of water. Heat the water to boiling; reduce to medium heat, cover, and steam the broccoli for 5 minutes or until just fork-tender and still bright green.

4. While the broccoli cooks, add onions and mushrooms to the skillet in which the meat was cooked and sauté for 1–2 minutes. Add 1½ cups broth, stirring to pick up any flavor bits off the bottom of the skillet.

5. In a separate bowl, combine the cornstarch and remaining broth and stir until smooth. Add broth mixture to the skillet and bring to a slow boil for 1 minute. Add meat back to the pan and keep warm. When ready to serve, place 1 cup cooked broccoli on each of 4 plates, top with ½ cup rice and a fourth of the steak and gravy. Sprinkle with parsley.

Yield: 4 servings
(serving size: about 1 cup steak and gravy, 1 cup broccoli, and ½ cup rice)

Nutrient Breakdown:
Calories 360

Fat 12g
(3.5g saturated fat)

Cholesterol 75mg

Sodium 400mg

Carbohydrate 32g

Fiber 5g

Protein 33g

Plate Plan choices:
1½ starches,
2 vegetables,
4 lean meats

Congrats! You made it through the toughest week of the Countdown to Your **BEST BODY!**

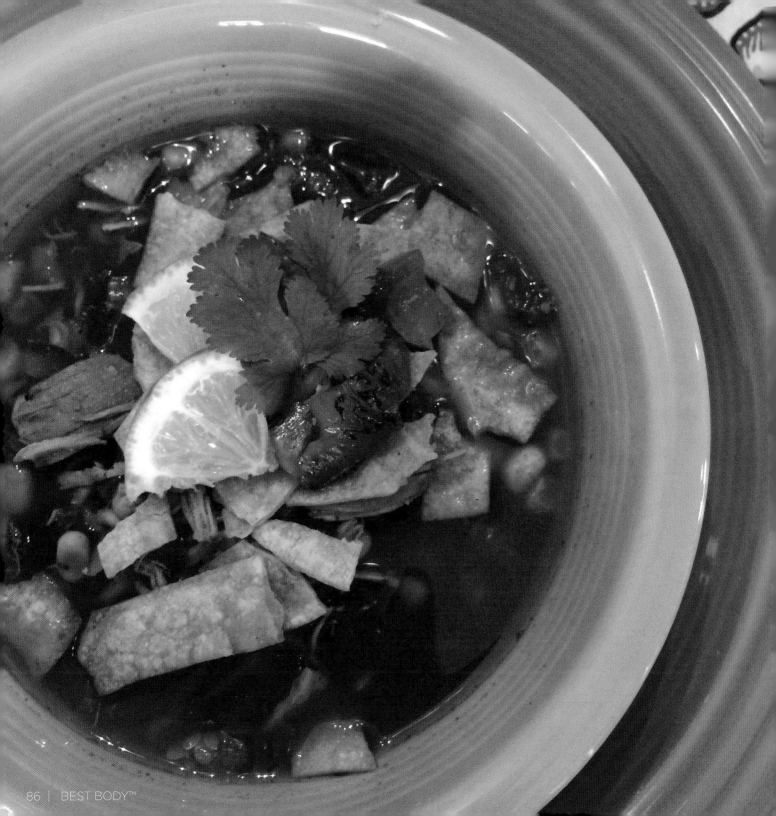

recipes & menu:
week two

recipes & menu: week two

> "The amount of our endurance is directly proportionate to the clarity of our vision."
> — RORY VADEN

menu key:

Lunch Leftovers

Pricey Meal

Quicker-Fix

Slow-Cooker

Club Favorite

Easy Meal

DAY 46
Mediterranean Mahi Mahi
Simple Sautéed Spinach
Suggested side: barley

DAY 45
Buffalo Chicken Pita Sandwich
Suggested sides: raw veggies with
Yogurt Ranch Dressing
steamed corn

DAY 44
Chicken Fiesta Soup
Avocado Salsa Topper

DAY 43
Cocoa-Spiced Pork
4-Ingredient Kale Salad
Suggested side: brown rice

DAY 42
Quinoa Salmon Patties
Oven Potato Fries
Suggested side: sugar snap peas and
carrots (steamable bag)

DAY 41
Penne Pasta Casserole
Sautéed Swiss Chard

DAY 40
Perfectly Filling Quinoa Lettuce Wraps
Sweet Protein Perfection

You have finished the toughest week of the Countdown! You should be proud of yourself! Now, let's review some of our kitchen and cooking basics:

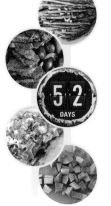

5 vegetable and fruit servings or more daily

4 cook-at-home meals weekly+

3 "Strategic Splurges" per week

2 meals from 1 (double recipes)

1 hour of pre-prep and planning time weekly

1. What should a "Best Body Breakfast" include?

2. Give an example of how you can get a minimum of five fruits and vegetables in a day.

3. Out of the seven dinner options we offer per week, how many do we suggest you make at home weekly? (Hint: See the 5-4-3-2-1 graphic.)

4. For strategy's sake, what time of day is the daily "Strong Snack" typically scheduled?

5. Do you know what your three "Strategic Splurges" for the week will be yet? Plan in advance to savor these and not let mindless splurges sneak up on you in the late moments of the evening.

6. After looking over the menu for the week, which recipes do you plan on doubling in order to get a second meal from them, or a "Lunch Leftover?"

7. For this week, what is imperative that you prepare during that hour of pre-prep and planning that we recommend?

8. A Best Body plate is half full of _____ at two meals per day, at least.

No answer key here... you've got all the answers in your book! Review the 5-4-3-2-1 graphic and commit this to memory. This time next year, you'll be glad you did when you are still sporting Your Best Body!

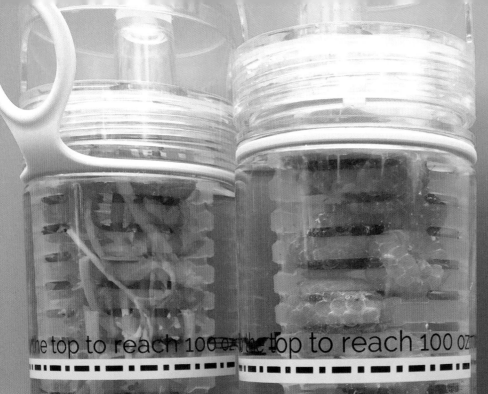
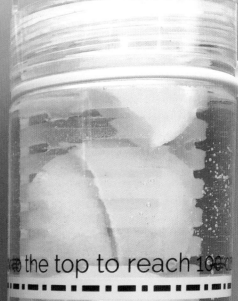
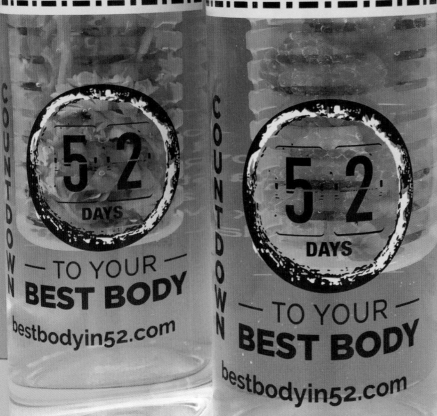
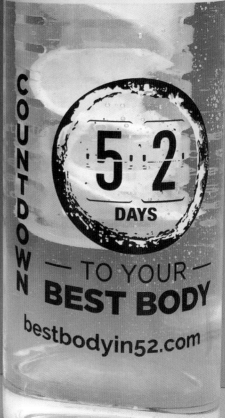

the top to reach 100 oz

COUNTDOWN

5 2 DAYS

— TO YOUR —
BEST BODY

bestbodyin52.com

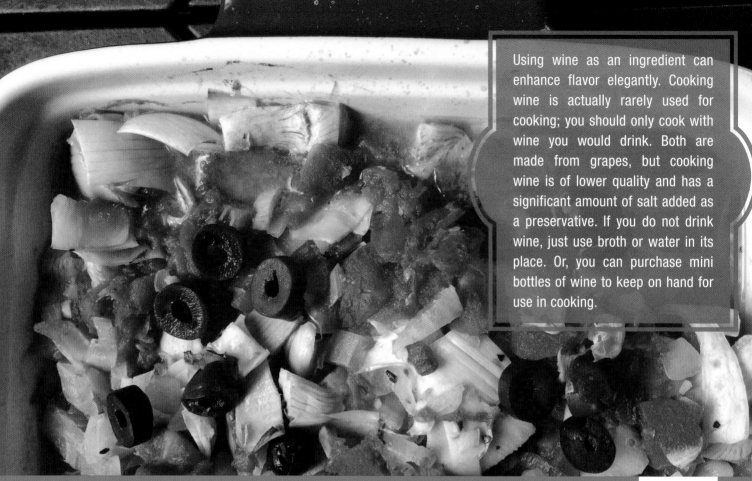

Using wine as an ingredient can enhance flavor elegantly. Cooking wine is actually rarely used for cooking; you should only cook with wine you would drink. Both are made from grapes, but cooking wine is of lower quality and has a significant amount of salt added as a preservative. If you do not drink wine, just use broth or water in its place. Or, you can purchase mini bottles of wine to keep on hand for use in cooking.

DAY 46

Pricey Meal

mediterranean mahi mahi

The sauce makes this recipe! It would work equally well with other firm white fish, such as halibut or cod, or even with chicken.

suggested side: barley

Total time: 30 minutes

To easily cut the stewed tomatoes, pour into a medium bowl and snip them with kitchen shears right in the bowl.

Canola oil cooking spray

4 4–5-ounce fresh or frozen mahi mahi fillets (soak or thaw in milk, if desired)

2 teaspoons extra-virgin olive oil

1 small onion, chopped (about 1 cup)

2 garlic cloves, minced

¼ cup dry white wine (such as chardonnay)

1 14.5-ounce can stewed tomatoes, chopped (reserve liquid)

½ teaspoon dried oregano

1 14-ounce can quartered artichoke hearts in water, drained

½ teaspoon Jane's Krazy Mixed-Up Salt

¼ teaspoon black pepper

¼ cup chopped black olives (optional garnish)

1. Preheat oven to 400°F. Cover a baking pan with aluminum foil (for easy clean up) and coat with cooking spray.

2. Pat fish dry with paper towels. Let the fish rest on the paper towels while you make the sauce. The paper towels will soak up any remaining liquid from the fish (the more liquid soaked up in this step the better, as it will allow the sauce to soak in and flavor the fish during cooking).

3. Coat a large nonstick skillet with cooking spray, add oil, and place over medium-high heat. Once hot, add onion and garlic. Cook until soft and translucent, 3–5 minutes.

4. Next, add the wine, tomatoes with reserved liquid, oregano, and artichokes. Mix well and simmer for about 5 minutes.

5. Arrange the fish in the prepared pan and sprinkle with salt and pepper. Pour the pan sauce over the fish and bake 12-15 minutes until it flakes with a fork. Sprinkle with olives before serving.

Yield: 4 servings
(serving size: 1 mah mahii fillet and ½–¾ cup sauce)

Nutrient Breakdown:
Calories 230

Fat 3.5g
(0.5g saturated fat,
140mg omega-3 fatty acids),

Cholesterol 50mg

Sodium 550mg

Carbohydrate 16g

Fiber 2g

Protein 27g

Plate Plan choices:
3 vegetables,
3 very lean meats

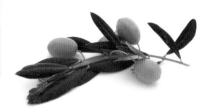

GROCERY LIST:

Onion (1)

Garlic cloves (2)

Mahi mahi fillets
(4 4–5-ounce fillets)

Canned
artichoke hearts
(1 14-ounce can)

Stewed tomatoes
(1 14.5-ounce can)

Dry white wine such
as chardonnay

Dried oregano

Jane's Krazy
Mixed-Up Salt

Black pepper

Black olives
(¼ cup, optional)

Extra-virgin
olive oil

Canola oil
cooking spray

Barley
(suggested side)

simple sautéed spinach

Total time: 10 minutes

This simple recipe is a great vegetable side for any night of the week. It can also be added to a grain bowl with protein for a quick, nutrient-rich lunch.

1 pound fresh baby spinach

1 tablespoon extra-virgin olive oil

4 cloves garlic, coarsely chopped

1/8 teaspoon salt

1/8 teaspoon black pepper

2 tablespoons lemon juice

GROCERY LIST:
Baby spinach
(16 ounces)

Garlic cloves (4)

Lemon or lemon juice
(2 tablespoons juice)

Salt

Black pepper

Extra-virgin olive oil

1. Rinse the spinach in a colander. Allow some of the water to remain on the spinach leaves (this will help it cook).

2. Add olive oil to a large pot or Dutch oven and place over medium heat. Once the oil is hot, add garlic and sauté for 30 seconds or until aromatic.

3. Add in spinach and stir to combine. Sprinkle with salt and pepper and cook for 3 minutes, until the spinach wilts. When ready to serve, drizzle with lemon juice.

Yield: 6 servings
(serving size: ½ cup)

Nutrient Breakdown:
Calories 60

Fat 2.5g
(2g monounsaturated fat)

Cholesterol 0mg

Sodium 170mg

Carbohydrate 9g

Fiber 4g

Protein 2g

Plate Plan choices:
2 vegetables, ½ fat

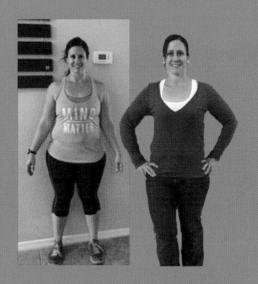

" After I had my two children, I knew I didn't want them to

go through some of the challenges that I had faced during

my childhood...I wanted to show them a healthy and active

lifestyle. Since I started about four months ago, I have lost 27

pounds and 11 inches (waist, hips, and thighs)."

—SANDRA, 35

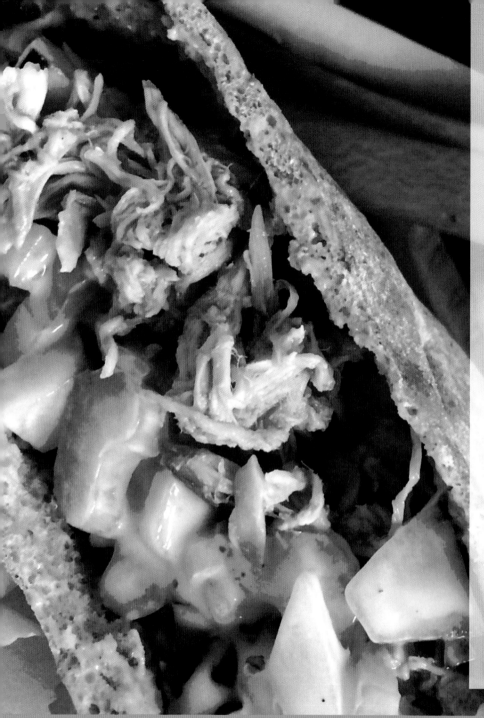

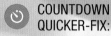 COUNTDOWN
QUICKER-FIX:

Option 1:
Use precooked chicken breast or pull the chicken off of a rotisserie chicken, using white meat first. You will need about 3 cups of shredded chicken. Place the butter and hot sauce in a medium-sized skillet over medium heat; add chicken and cook until it is heated through. Add more hot sauce if desired, using the least amount needed, as the sauce and the rotisserie chicken are both high in sodium. Build sandwiches as directed, or simply layer cucumbers in the pita bread and top with yogurt-based ranch dressing.

Option 2:
We also tested this recipe using the slow cooker, which can be a great alternate cooking method, depending on the flow of your day. This turned out just right: add the chicken breasts, hot sauce and butter to the slow cooker, swish around to coat chicken in the sauce, and cook on high for 4 hours. When done, shred the chicken with a fork while still in the slow cooker, mixing it with the sauce. Serve as directed.

*To seed a cucumber, cut the cucumber in half lengthwise, then scoop or scrape the seeds out with a spoon and discard. This keeps the cucumbers from adding too much liquid.

Hands-on time: 20 minutes
Total time: 35 minutes, if you prepare the cucumber topping while the chicken is in the oven

Slow-Cooker
Optional

buffalo chicken pita sandwiches

Quicker-Fix   Lunch Leftovers

This is a fun recipe that can be used many ways. During recipe testing, we shared the extra chicken over salad greens and pita wedges with interns for a great "Lunch Leftover." It was delicious! Go ahead and plan to make extra for sandwiches or salads (packing the pita separately to prevent it from getting soggy).

suggested sides:
raw vegetables
and steamed corn

Canola oil cooking spray

1 pound boneless, skinless chicken breasts, trimmed of fat

3 tablespoons hot sauce, divided

2 tablespoons yogurt-based ranch dressing (such as Bolthouse Farms)

½ cucumber, seeded* and chopped

1 stalk celery, finely chopped

1 tablespoon butter

2 whole-wheat pita rounds

Additional celery, cucumber and carrot slices for serving on the side

1. Preheat the oven to 400°F .
2. Coat a baking dish with cooking spray and arrange the chicken in the dish. Pour 1 tablespoon hot sauce over the chicken and turn the chicken to coat with sauce. Cover the pan with aluminum foil and seal the edges tightly. Bake for 20–25 minutes or until done. Chicken is done when the internal temperature registers 165°F on a meat thermometer.
3. While the chicken cooks, combine the cucumber and celery with 2 tablespoons ranch dressing.
4. Once the chicken is done, remove it and chop or shred. Return the chicken to the baking dish and add the butter and the remaining 2 tablespoons of hot sauce. Stir to combine. Return the pan back to the oven for a few minutes until butter melts and sauce is heated.
5. To serve, place pita bread on a microwavable plate, cover with a very slightly damp paper towel, and microwave for 10 seconds. Cut each pita in half and stuff with chicken and cucumber mixture.

Yield: 4 servings
(½ pita round, ½ cup chicken mixture, and ¼ cup cucumber salad)

Nutrient Breakdown:
Calories 260

Fat 8g (2.5g saturated fat)

Cholesterol 80mg

Sodium 680mg

Carbohydrate 21g

Fiber 3g

Protein 28g

Plate Plan choices:
1 starch, ½ vegetable, 4 very lean meats, 1 fat

GROCERY LIST:
Cucumber (1)

Celery

Whole-wheat pita rounds (2)

Boneless, skinless chicken breasts (1 pound), or use 1 rotisserie chicken

Hot sauce

Greek yogurt-based ranch dressing (Bolthouse Farms)

Butter

Canola oil cooking spray

Corn (suggested side)

Fresh celery, cucumber, carrots, and red pepper strips (suggested side)

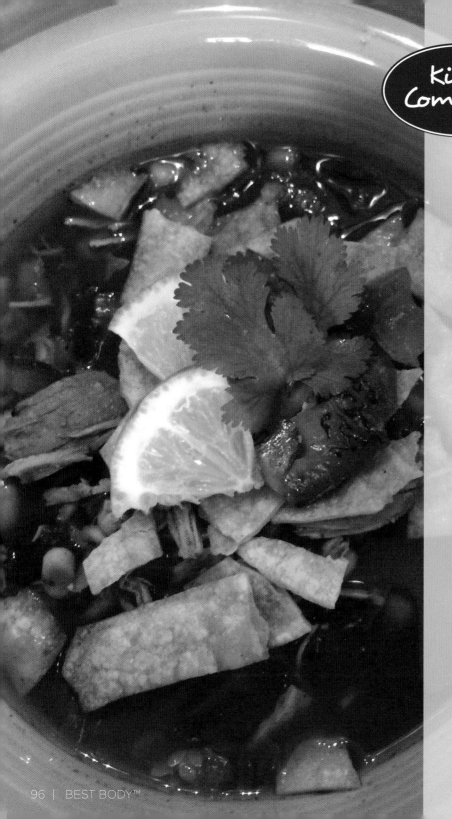

Store-bought broth is one of my secret cooking weapons. I have this in my pantry at all times and recommend you do the same. It is lovely to use when cooking whole grains or for a quick sauté of vegetables when you need to add a little moisture to the pan without adding extra oil. In our recipes, we use either reduced sodium or unsalted broth. When unsalted broth is called for, use it instead of reduced-sodium broth. We chose that sodium level to help keep the total sodium in the recipe down.

Suggestions:

- Buy the best quality you can afford (it is used for adding flavor to food, so quality is important).

- Purchase broth in the 32-ounce size (it is more economical than buying smaller containers).

- If you do not use the entire container of broth, either refrigerate it for up to 7 days or freeze the leftovers. I freeze mine in ice cube trays and then pop the cubes out and keep them in a plastic zip-top freezer bag so I can pull a cube out whenever I need some.

Slow-Cooker

chicken fiesta soup

Hands-on time: 15 minutes
Total time: 8 hours and 15 minutes

Lunch Leftovers

Club Favorite

This Mexican-inspired slow-cooker soup is sure to please the whole family. It's great for a weeknight meal and is equally nice for a weekend fiesta. The Avocado Salsa Topper (recipe follows) is a perfect pairing, but if time doesn't allow, diced avocado can be added as a topping when serving the soup.

2 teaspoons cumin

1½ tablespoons chili powder

1 teaspoon dried oregano

1 pound boneless, skinless chicken breasts

1 14.5-ounce can diced fire-roasted tomatoes

2 tablespoons tomato paste

1 large onion, chopped (about 2 cups)

1 medium zucchini, chopped (about 1½ cups)

1 12-ounce bag frozen corn, thawed

1 4-ounce can diced green chilies

3 garlic cloves, minced

1 cup water

4 cups unsalted chicken broth

¼ teaspoon black pepper

1 bay leaf

6 corn tortillas

Canola oil cooking spray

Cilantro

Lime wedges

1. Combine the first 3 seasonings in a bowl and set one teaspoon aside for the tortillas.

2. Place the next 12 ingredients (chicken through bay leaf) and the mixed seasonings from step 1 in the slow cooker. Cook on low for 6–8 hours or on high for 3–4 hours.

3. Once the soup is done, remove the chicken breasts and bay leaf from the soup. Shred the chicken and add it back to the soup. Discard the bay leaf.

4. To prepare the tortillas, preheat the oven to 425°F. Cut the tortillas into strips using a pizza cutter (or clean kitchen shears). Begin at one side and cut almost all the way to the other side of the tortilla (this will make them easy to flip over and break apart after cooking). Place tortillas on the baking sheet, spray each side with cooking spray, and sprinkle with the reserved seasoning mixture. Bake for 3–4 minutes on each side or until crisp (watch closely, as they can burn easily). Break them into strips.

5. Top the soup with tortilla strips, cilantro, lime wedges and Avocado Salsa Topper.

Yield: 6 servings
(serving size: 1¾ cup soup and 1 tortilla)

Nutrient Breakdown:
Calories 290

Fat 4.5g
(1g saturated fat)

Cholesterol 50mg

Sodium 550mg

Carbohydrate 38g

Fiber 6g

Protein 23g

Plate Plan choices:
1½ starches,
2 vegetables,
3 very lean meats,
1 fat

GROCERY LIST:

Onion (1 large)	Corn tortillas (6)	Unsalted chicken broth	Black pepper
Zucchini (1 medium)	Diced fire-roasted tomatoes (1 14.5-ounce can)	Frozen corn (12 ounces)	Bay leaves
Garlic cloves (3)			Canola oil cooking spray
Boneless, skinless chicken breasts (1 pound)	Tomato paste	Cumin	Cilantro
	Diced green chilies (4-ounce can)	Chili powder	Lime, for wedges
		Dried oregano	

avocado salsa topper

Total time: 10 minutes

Avocados and lime juice are natural garnishes for Mexican cuisine. This recipe is also great as a baked potato topper: just add some grilled chicken, and you have a quick lunch.

1 ripe avocado, chopped

1 medium tomato, chopped

1 garlic clove, minced or pounded with mortar and pestle

1 tablespoon lime juice

2 tablespoons finely diced red onion

2 teaspoons diced jalapeño (jarred or fresh)

1/8 teaspoon salt

1/4 cup chopped fresh cilantro

1/4 cup Mexican crumbled cheese (queso fresco) or feta cheese

GROCERY LIST:
Avocado (1)

Tomato (1 medium)

Garlic clove (1)

Lime or lime juice (1 tablespoon)

Red onion (1 small)

Jalapeño

Fresh cilantro

Mexican crumbling cheese such as queso fresco or feta cheese (1/4 cup)

Salt

This is a crowd-pleaser as a dip with pita chips, too (See Day 28 for our homemade Pita Chips recipe).

1. In a medium bowl, stir all of the ingredients together gently. Garnish with additional cilantro if desired.

Yield: 6 servings
(serving size: 2 tablespoons)

Nutrient Breakdown:
Calories 70

Fat 5g (1g saturated fat)

Cholesterol 0mg

Sodium 60mg

Carbohydrate 5g

Fiber 3g

Protein 1g

Plate Plan choices:
1 vegetable, 1 fat

Easy Meal

cocoa-spiced pork

Total time: 20 minutes
suggested side: brown rice
(precooked, if available)

Quicker-Fix

Lunch Leftovers

The seasoning combinations of this rub combine to provide warmth and a mellow flavor that is unique and pairs nicely with rice or potatoes. You may want to double the recipe to use for "Lunch Leftovers."

Rub
1 tablespoon chili powder

1 tablespoon cocoa powder

½ teaspoon ground coffee

¼ teaspoon cinnamon

1 teaspoon Jane's Krazy Mixed-Up Salt

Pork
4 4-ounce center-cut loin chops, trimmed of fat

Canola oil cooking spray

1 tablespoon canola oil

1 medium onion, chopped

1 cup reduced-sodium chicken broth

1 tablespoon cornstarch

¼ cup water

1. Combine rub ingredients in a large plastic zip-top bag. Add pork to the bag, zip, and shake to coat the pork with seasonings.

2. Coat a large nonstick skillet with cooking spray and place over medium-high heat, and then add the oil. Once hot, swirl to coat pan; add pork and cook 4–6 minutes on each side until nice and brown. Transfer pork to a plate and tent with foil.

3. Reduce heat to medium and add onions to the skillet. Allow them to cook for 30–60 seconds. Add the broth to the pan and stir to get the brown bits from the bottom of the pan.

4. Combine cornstarch and water, add to the pan, and boil for 1 minute or until thick. Add the pork back to the pan, cover, and cook until done (4–6 minutes or until the internal temperature of the pork reaches 145°F on a meat thermometer). Serve gravy with the pork.

Yield: 4 servings
(serving size: 1 pork chop and ½ cup gravy)

Nutrient Breakdown:
Calories 180

Fat 10g
(2g saturated fat)

Cholesterol 60mg

Sodium 480mg

Carbohydrate 6g

Fiber 1g

Protein 19g

Plate Plan choices:
½ starch, 3 lean meats

GROCERY LIST:

Onion (1 medium)

Center-cut loin chops (4 4-ounce chops)

Reduced-sodium chicken broth

Chili powder

Cocoa powder

Ground coffee

Cinnamon

Jane's Krazy Mixed-Up Salt

Cornstarch

Canola oil

Canola oil cooking spray

 COUNTDOWN QUICKER-FIX:

Your evening will be simplified if you have frozen pork loin on hand from last week's Garlic Pork Loin recipe. Simply make the rub as directed in step 1, then rub it evenly on 4 slices of cooked pork loin (2–3 ounces each). Follow the directions as listed, keeping in mind that you will only need to sear the pork for about 2–3 minutes in step 2.

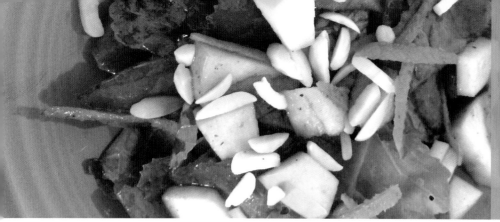

To Massage Kale:

Combine clean, bite-sized mature kale and 1 tablespoon of dressing in a large bowl. Gently massage the kale, squeezing it through your fingers for 1–2 minutes. It will become shiny, velvet-like, and will decrease in volume by half. Drain out any accumulated juices.

4-ingredient kale salad

Total time: 10 minutes (if using mature kale)

Club Favorite

Kale is more and more available at supermarkets and farmer's markets these days. Baby kale leaves are tender enough to eat raw in salads. If you can only find mature kale, you can still eat a delicious kale salad by massaging the kale. Sounds a little strange, but the technique is simple.

1 medium Granny Smith apple, skin on, cored and roughly chopped

3–4 tablespoons balsamic vinaigrette (such as Newman's Own)

1 5-ounce package baby kale (about 6 cups packed)

½ cup shredded carrots (or one large carrot, shredded)

2 tablespoons toasted almonds or ¼ cup shredded Parmesan cheese (from refrigerated section)

1. Combine apples with 1 tablespoon vinaigrette to prevent browning.

2. Toss baby kale, apples, and carrots together in a medium bowl. Add dressing one tablespoon at a time in an effort to use the least amount necessary on the salad. (If using massaged kale, little to no additional dressing is needed.)

3. Top with toasted almonds or Parmesan cheese when ready to serve.

Yield: 4 servings
(serving size: 1¾ cups salad and ½ tablespoon almonds or Parmesan cheese)

Nutrient Breakdown:
Calories 80

Fat 3.5g (0g saturated fat)

Cholesterol 0mg

Sodium 110mg

Carbohydrate 11g

Fiber 2g

Protein 2g

Plate Plan choices:
1½ vegetables, 1 fat

GROCERY LIST:
Granny Smith apple (1)

Shredded carrots or one large carrot (½ cup shredded)

Baby or mature kale (5 ounces or about 6 cups, packed)

Almonds (2 tablespoons) or shredded Parmesan cheese (¼ cup)

Balsamic vinaigrette (Newman's Own recommended)

quinoa salmon patties

Total time: 30 minutes

Lunch Leftovers

Salmon is a wonderful source of omega-3 fatty acids. Canned salmon is a convenient and economical way of adding more omega-3s to your diet. Those who don't enjoy traditionally prepared fish may be willing to try it this way. Sohaillaʼs kids love to have leftover salmon patties on a bun for lunch: consider doubling this recipe for "Lunch Leftovers."

Canola oil cooking spray

1 tablespoon extra-virgin olive oil, divided

1 bunch green onions, whites and greens chopped and separated

1 stalk celery, chopped

Zest of half a lemon (about 1 teaspoon)

2 teaspoons lemon juice

2 teaspoons chopped fresh dill (or ¾ teaspoon dried dill)

1 15-ounce can of salmon

½ cup cooked quinoa

2 teaspoons Dijon mustard

1 egg plus 2 egg whites

½ teaspoon black pepper

Lemon wedges (optional)

1. Coat a large nonstick skillet with cooking spray, place over medium heat and add ½ teaspoon oil. Once hot, add the white part of the onions and celery. Stir and cook until the celery is soft (about 2 minutes). Remove from pan and allow the vegetables to cool.

2. Add ½ of the onion tops to the bowl of a food processor with the lemon zest, juice and dill. Pulse the onions for 6 1-second pulses until onions are minced.

3. Drain, debone and remove the skin from the salmon. Place the salmon in a large bowl, break it up with a fork, and add it to the food processor. Add the quinoa, mustard, and celery mixture to the food processor and pulse until a dough begins to form and ingredients are mixed (about 10 pulses).

4. In the same bowl used for the salmon, whisk the eggs, egg whites and pepper with a fork. Add the salmon mixture to the eggs and mix well. Divide the salmon into 4 equal patties and set aside.

5. Add the remaining 2½ teaspoons of oil to the same pan used for the celery and place over medium heat. Once the oil is hot, add the patties and cook until golden brown (about 3 minutes). Carefully flip and cook on the other side until heated through (2–3 minutes). Serve with lemon wedges, if desired.

Yield: 4 servings
(serving size: 1 salmon patty)

Nutrient Breakdown:
Calories 240

Fat 14g (2.5g saturated fat, ~750mg omega-3 fatty acids)

Cholesterol 70mg

Sodium 480mg

Carbohydrate 7g

Fiber 1g

Protein 19g

Plate Plan choices:
½ starch, 2½ lean meats, 1 fat

GROCERY LIST:
Green onions (1 bunch)

Celery

Fresh or dried dill

Lemon (2 needed for the zest, juice, and wedges for serving)

Salmon (1 15-ounce can)

Quinoa (½ cup cooked)

Eggs (3)

Dijon mustard

Extra-virgin olive oil

Canola oil cooking spray

Black pepper

Sugar snap peas and carrots (suggested side)

oven potato fries

Sometimes you just want some fries… better served here than at a restaurant in a bottomless basket! Potatoes are actually a great source of potassium, and with the skin, they have a bit of fiber, too. Moderation is key!

Canola oil cooking spray

1 pound baking potatoes, scrubbed (about 2 medium)

1 tablespoon canola oil

½ teaspoon paprika

¼ teaspoon black pepper

½ teaspoon salt, divided

GROCERY LIST:
Baking potatoes
(2 medium)

Paprika

Salt

Black pepper

Canola oil

Canola oil cooking spray

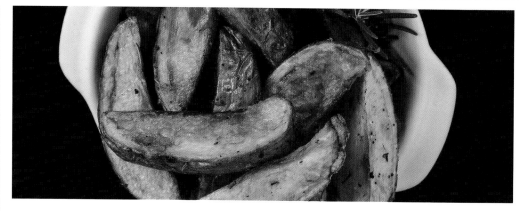

1. Preheat oven to 450°F. Cover a baking sheet with aluminum foil (for easy clean up) and spray with cooking spray.

2. Cut the potatoes in half lengthwise. With the cut side facing the cutting board, cut each half into quarters lengthwise. Turn each quarter on its side so the newly cut side is on the cutting board, and cut in half lengthwise, creating approximately ½-inch thick fries. Repeat until all the potatoes are cut into fries.

3. Make sure potatoes are fairly dry by placing them on a paper towel-lined plate once cut (drying the potatoes helps the oil coat them better). Add potatoes to a large bowl and toss with oil, paprika, pepper, and ¼ teaspoon salt.

4. Place in a single layer on the baking sheet and bake for 20 minutes. Stir or flip the fries halfway through the cooking time. Sprinkle with remaining ¼ teaspoon salt.

Yield: 4 servings
(serving size: about 8-10 fries)

Nutrient Breakdown:
Calories 120

Fat 3.5g (0g saturated fat, 2g monounsaturated fat),

Cholesterol 0mg

Sodium 300mg

Carbohydrate 20g

Fiber 1g

Protein 2g

Plate Plan choices:
1 starch, 1 fat

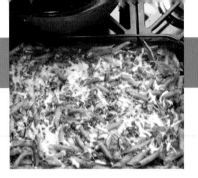

penne pasta casserole

Lunch Leftovers

Club Favorite

This Best Body Club favorite is easy, tasty, and healthy: a win-win-win! The perfect comfort food!

Hands-on time: 30 minutes
Total time: 45 minutes

8 ounces uncooked whole-wheat penne pasta (generous 3 cups dry)

12 ounces all-natural chicken sausage, casings removed (such as Al Fresco all natural sweet Italian-style chicken sausage)

1 green bell pepper, chopped (1 cup)

1 large zucchini, chopped

1 small onion, chopped (1 cup)

2 teaspoons Italian seasoning

½ teaspoon garlic powder

1 28-ounce can tomato puree or pasta sauce

1 cup part-skim mozzarella cheese, divided

Canola oil cooking spray

3 tablespoons grated Parmesan cheese

1. Preheat the oven to 350°F.
2. Cook the pasta in a large pot 2 minutes less than indicated on the package instructions, (ideally, the pasta should be just slightly undercooked, as it will continue cooking in the oven).
3. Meanwhile, in a nonstick skillet, cook sausage over medium heat, breaking it up as it cooks. Once the sausage is cooked, add the pepper, zucchini, and onion and sauté until the onion is translucent, about 5–7 minutes. Add the seasonings and sauce and stir until combined.
4. Once the pasta is cooked, drain it and return it to the pot. Add the sauce to the pasta pot with ¾ cup of mozzarella cheese, stirring to combine.
5. Transfer the pasta to a 9x13-inch baking dish that has been sprayed with cooking spray and bake for 10 minutes. Top with the remaining ¼ cup mozzarella and Parmesan cheeses. Bake for an additional 5 minutes until golden on top.

Choose sauce with the least sodium and sugar.

Yield: 8 servings
(serving size: 1½ cups)

Nutrient Breakdown:
Calories 280

Fat 9g (3.5g saturated fat)

Cholesterol 45mg

Sodium 410mg

Carbohydrate 32g

Fiber 7g

Protein 19g

Plate Plan choices:
2 starches, 1 vegetable, 2 medium-fat meats

GROCERY LIST:
Green pepper (1)

Onion (1 small)

Zucchini (1 large)

Chicken or turkey sausage (12 ounces)

Whole-wheat penne pasta (8 ounces)

Tomato puree or pasta sauce (28 ounces)

Part-skim mozzarella cheese (1 cup)

Grated Parmesan cheese

Italian seasoning

Garlic powder

Canola oil cooking spray

sautéed swiss chard

Swiss chard is a great way to begin adding greens to your diet because it is fairly mild in taste. Feel free to buy pre-chopped Swiss chard to minimize prep time. Enjoy!

1 bunch of Swiss chard
(about 1 pound)

Canola oil cooking spray

2 teaspoons extra-virgin olive oil

½ onion chopped (about ½ cup)

2 cloves garlic, minced

4 teaspoons grated
Parmesan cheese

Broth or water as needed

Lemon juice or wedges

GROCERY LIST:
Swiss chard
(1 bunch or about 1 pound)

Onion

Garlic cloves (2)

Lemon (1) or lemon juice

Grated Parmesan cheese

Broth

Extra-virgin olive oil

Canola oil cooking spray

1. Rinse the Swiss chard well in a colander or salad spinner (make sure all the dirt is rinsed away). Shake the excess water off. Stack the leaves, then cut the stems off and set both aside. Next, with leaves still stacked, cut the leaves in half along the stem line. Then, slice them across in 1-inch pieces. Cut the stems into ½-inch pieces, discarding the bottom piece.

2. Place a large nonstick skillet or Dutch oven over medium heat, coat with cooking spray and add oil. When the oil is hot, add onion, garlic, and chard stems and sauté 2 minutes.

3. Add the Swiss chard greens to the pan. You may have to add greens a little at a time: as the greens wilt, there will be more room in the pan for the remaining greens. Cook greens for about 4 minutes until they are wilted and tender (add broth or water to pan as needed to facilitate cooking).

4. Serve with a squeeze of lemon juice and Parmesan cheese.

Yield: 4 servings
(serving size: 1 cup)

Nutrient Breakdown:
Calories 60

Fat 3g (0.5g saturated fat)

Cholesterol 0mg

Sodium 270mg

Carbohydrate 7g

Fiber 2g

Protein 3g

Plate Plan choices:
2 vegetables, ½ fat

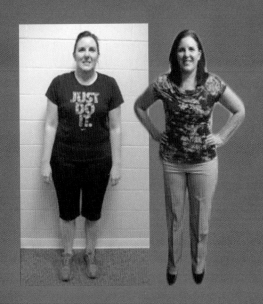

❝ I honestly did not think I would see the the

changes that I have! I am down 14 pounds and 8

inches in such a short amount of time! The recipes

are great and will stay a part of my weekly menus.

—SHAWNA, 45

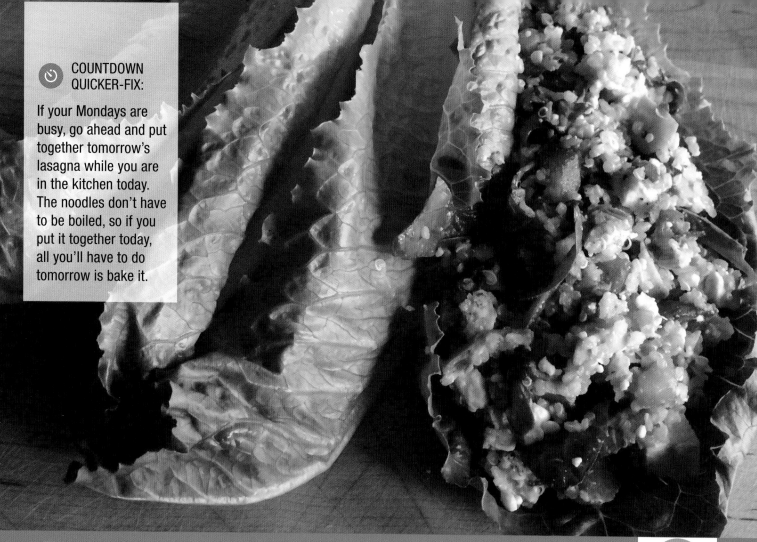

⏱ **COUNTDOWN QUICKER-FIX:**

If your Mondays are busy, go ahead and put together tomorrow's lasagna while you are in the kitchen today. The noodles don't have to be boiled, so if you put it together today, all you'll have to do tomorrow is bake it.

DAY 40

Easy Meal

perfectly filling quinoa lettuce wraps

Lunch Leftovers

Club Favorite

This recipe is a Best Body Club favorite not only because of its fabulous taste, but also because of its versatility. We suggest doubling this recipe. The wrap filling is perfect the next day in a mason jar when dashing out for lunch. Just don't forget a spoon or fork.

Total time: 30 minutes

1 cup water

½ cup quinoa (or 2 cups precooked quinoa)

2 medium tomatoes, chopped

2 cups packed fresh spinach, coarsely chopped

5 green onions, chopped (about ½ cup)

1 avocado, peeled and cut in small chunks

¾ cup crumbled feta cheese (3 ounces)

½ teaspoon Jane's Krazy Mixed-Up Salt or Cavender's Greek Seasoning

8 ounces chopped cooked chicken (optional)

1 tablespoon lime juice (juice of ½ lime)

8 large romaine lettuce leaves (for wraps)

1. Bring water to a boil in a medium-sized pot and add quinoa. Cover and reduce heat. Simmer for 15 minutes, or until the water has been absorbed.

2. While chopping the vegetables, cool the quinoa in a shallow baking dish in the refrigerator.

3. Place vegetables in a large bowl.

4. Add chilled quinoa to vegetables and toss. Add crumbled feta cheese, seasoning, and chicken (if desired). Squeeze lime juice over the lettuce wrap filling and mix gently.

5. Scoop about a cup of quinoa mix into each romaine lettuce leaf to make lettuce wraps.

GROCERY LIST:

Tomatoes (2 medium)	Avocado (1)	Quinoa
Fresh spinach (2 cups)	Lime juice (1 tablespoon)	Feta cheese (3 ounces)
Green onions (5)	Cooked chicken (8 ounces, optional)	Jane's Krazy Mixed-Up Salt or Cavender's Greek Seasoning
Romaine lettuce (8 large leaves)		

Yield: 4 servings
(serving size: 2 lettuce wraps)

Nutrient Breakdown:
(with chicken):
Calories 240 (300)

Fat 12g (13g),
3.5g (4g saturated fat)

Cholesterol 10mg (45mg)

Sodium 410mg

Carbohydrate 23g

Fiber 7g

Protein 9g (20g)

Plate Plan choices:
1 starch, 2 vegetables, 1 very lean meat, 2 fats

Sohailla Says

I sometimes put this in a mason jar instead of a romaine wrap and take it on the go. We tried it with our 3 kids at the beach, so we didn't have to leave for lunch or deal with sandy hands on sandwiches. Mission accomplished! It's great with chicken, but you won't miss the meat if you go without it in this dish.

sweet protein perfection

Total time: 8 minutes

Quicker-Fix

Need a quick dessert that provides a little protein punch? Then this is for you. You can also use it as a "Strong Snack." Feel free to change the yogurt flavor or the type of berries. For example, frozen wild blueberries are a great substitute if strawberries are not in season.

1 5.3-ounce container lemon-flavored Greek yogurt

⅓ cup low-fat ricotta cheese

1 teaspoon lemon juice

½ teaspoon lemon zest

¼ teaspoon almond extract

¼ cup slivered almonds, toasted

2 cups sliced strawberries

GROCERY LIST:
Strawberries (2 cups sliced)

Lemon (1 for juice and zest)

Lemon-flavored Greek yogurt (5.3-ounce container)

Low-fat ricotta cheese (⅓ cup)

Almond extract (¼ teaspoon)

Slivered almonds (¼ cup)

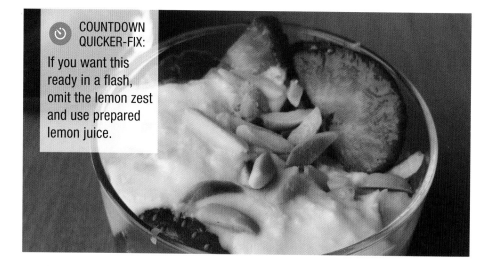

COUNTDOWN QUICKER-FIX:
If you want this ready in a flash, omit the lemon zest and use prepared lemon juice.

1. Combine the first five ingredients (yogurt through extract) in a medium bowl and mix until combined.
2. When ready to serve, top berries with Greek yogurt and almonds.

Yield: 4 servings
(servings size: ½ cup berries, 3 tablespoons yogurt mixture, and 1 tablespoon almonds)

Nutrient Breakdown:
Calories 120

Fat 4.5g (1g saturated fat)

Cholesterol 5mg

Sodium 45mg

Carbohydrate 13g

Added sugar 3g (from presweetened yogurt)

Fiber 3g

Protein 8g

Plate Plan choices:
½ milk, ½ fruit, 1 fat

Kim's Comment

Cookbooks have a lot more than recipes to offer: they are a wealth of information. Incorporating ricotta cheese into Greek yogurt for a texture and protein boost is something I learned recently when reading a cookbook by another RDN. Share something you have learned so far from reading this cookbook on the Best Body in 52 Facebook page!

recipes & menu:
week three

> " Let food be your medicine, and your medicine be your food."
> —HIPPOCRATES

menu key:

Lunch Leftovers

Pricey Meal

Quicker-Fix

Slow-Cooker

Club Favorite

Easy Meal

DAY 39
Best-Ever Spinach Lasagna

Suggested sides: green salad
Italian bread

DAY 38
Salmon with Salsa Verde

Cilantro-Lime Rice

Suggested side: squash and zucchini

DAY 37
Steakhouse Chicken

Cuban-Style Black Beans

Roasted Asparagus with Garlic
and Lemon

DAY 36
Planned-Over Best-Ever Spinach Lasagna

Green Beans with Toasted Almonds

DAY 35
Jerk Fish Tacos with Pineapple Salsa

Suggested side: green salad

DAY 34
All-American Backyard Burger

Refreshing Rainbow Salad

DAY 33
Dad's Oven-Roasted Chicken
with Vegetables

Suggested side: steamed broccoli

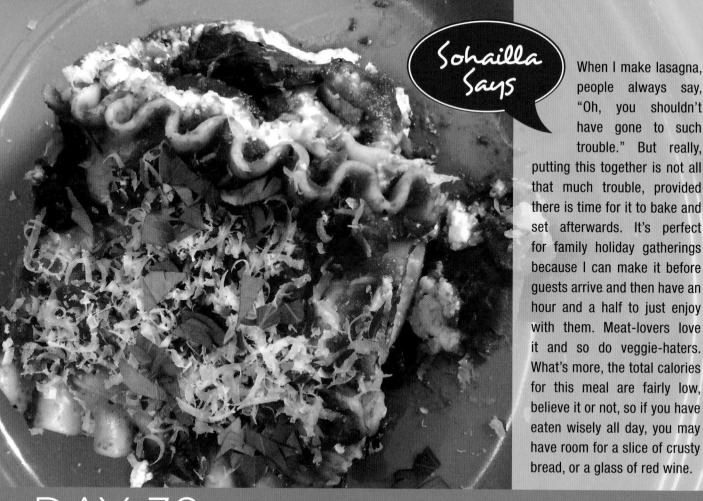

DAY 39

best-ever spinach lasagna

Total time: 1 hour 50 minutes
(30 minutes prep plus bake/set time)

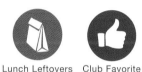

Lunch Leftovers   Club Favorite

This is delicious and provides two veggie servings in just one serving of lasagna! If you've always enjoyed meat-lover's lasagna, give this one a try… it might just make a veggie-lover out of you! This makes a lot, so go ahead and invite loved ones over to eat, or save half of the lasagna for a "planned-over" (scheduled on Day 36).

suggested sides: green salad and one slice of crusty Italian bread

1 16-ounce container low-fat cottage cheese

1 16-ounce container nonfat cottage cheese

2 cups part-skim mozzarella cheese, divided

¼ cup Parmesan Cheese

2 eggs, beaten

1 teaspoon dried basil

1½ 28-ounce jars of pasta sauce

1 14.5-ounce can stewed tomatoes, juice reserved

1 14.5-ounce can diced tomatoes, juice drained

6 packed cups slightly torn fresh spinach (5 ounces)

½ teaspoon Greek seasoning (such as Cavendar's)

4 garlic cloves, minced

1 9-ounce box oven-ready lasagna noodles (12–16 noodles)

1. Preheat oven to 425°F.

2. In a large bowl, combine cottage cheeses, mozzarella cheese, Parmesan cheese, eggs and dried basil. Mix well.

3. In another large bowl, combine pasta sauce, stewed tomatoes with juice, diced tomatoes without juice, garlic, spinach and Greek seasoning. Mix well.

4. In the bottom of a 9x13-inch baking pan, spread the following evenly:
   · 1½ cups sauce
   · 4–5 noodles, spaced across the sauce
   · ½ of the cheese mixture
   · ⅓ of the remaining pasta sauce
   · 4 noodles
   · all the remaining cheese mixture
   · ½ of the remaining pasta sauce
   · 4 noodles
   · all of the remaining pasta sauce

5. Wrap the lasagna tightly with a double layer of foil (spray the layer of foil that comes in contact with the food with cooking spray to keep it from sticking). Bake for 60 minutes. Uncover, top with the remaining mozzarella cheese, and return to the oven for 5 minutes to melt the cheese. After 5 minutes, turn the oven broiler on and standby watching as it cooks 6–8 inches under the broiler, removing it from the oven just when it begins to brown. Allow the lasagna to set for 30–40 minutes before cutting into 12 equal pieces.

Yield: 12 servings
(serving size: 1 piece)

Nutrient Breakdown:
Calories 270

Fat 8g (4g saturated fat)

Cholesterol 50mg

Sodium 290mg

Carbohydrate 30g

Fiber 3g

Protein 16g

Plate Plan choices:
1 starch, 2 vegetables, 2 medium-fat meats

" Delicious! Everyone we serve it to wants the recipe, especially when they hear how it's quick to prepare and just 270 calories."

—ALLAN, 71

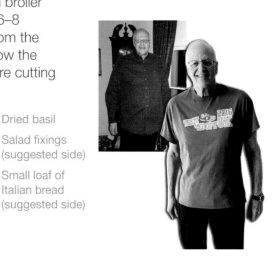

GROCERY LIST:
Fresh spinach, chopped (6 ounces or 4 cups packed)

Garlic cloves (4)

Oven-ready lasagna noodles (9-ounce box)

Spaghetti sauce (2 28-ounce jars)

Stewed tomatoes (14.5-ounce can)

Diced tomatoes (14.5-ounce can)

Low-fat cottage cheese (16-ounce container)

Nonfat cottage cheese (16-ounce container)

Reduced-fat Parmesan cheese

Part-skim mozzarella cheese (2 cups)

Eggs (2)

Greek seasoning (such as Cavendar's)

Dried basil

Salad fixings (suggested side)

Small loaf of Italian bread (suggested side)

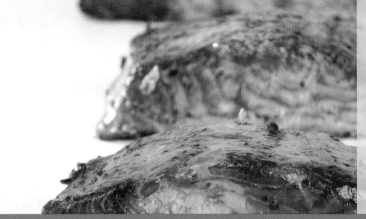

When you see how easy it is to make your own salsa verde, you will be glad you did: it tastes so good and fresh. Feel free to make this recipe spicier by adding additional peppers or hotter peppers. Leftover sauce can be served over baked chicken or rice, or in tacos. (If you don't have time to home-make the salsa verde, be sure to choose the jarred one with the least sodium, as salsa verde from a jar is very high in sodium.)

Kim's Comment

DAY 38

Easy Meal

salmon with salsa verde

You will want to serve this salmon with something that will get good mileage out of the delightful green sauce; we recommend Cilantro-Lime Rice.

Hands-on time: 10 minutes   Total time: 20 minutes

suggested side: sautéed squash and zucchini

Canola oil cooking spray

1 jalapeño pepper, cut in half and seeds removed

1 poblano pepper, cut in half and seeds removed

4 tomatillos, papery skins removed and cut in half

¼ cup packed fresh cilantro

4 4-ounce salmon fillets, Pacific wild-caught preferred (soak or thaw in milk, if desired)

1 teaspoon Jane's Krazy Mixed-Up Salt

Lime wedges (optional but delicious)

1. Preheat broiler. Line a baking sheet with aluminum foil (for easy clean up) and spray with cooking spray.

2. Place the peppers, tomatillos, and cilantro in a blender with about 2 tablespoons water. Blend until smooth and set aside.

3. Place salmon (skin side down) on the prepared baking sheet and sprinkle with seasoning salt. Broil 6 inches from the heat for 4–6 minutes on each side, depending on the thickness of the fish. When turning the salmon at the halfway point, remove the skin easily by sliding a spatula under the skin and return to oven. Serve with sauce and lime wedges.

Yield: 4 servings
(serving size: 1 fillet)

Nutrient Breakdown:
Calories 180

Fat 8g (1g saturated fat, 1200mg omega-3 fatty acids)

Cholesterol 60mg

Sodium 340mg

Carbohydrate 4g

Fiber 2g

Protein 23g

Plate Plan choices:
3 lean meats, 1 vegetable

GROCERY LIST:
Jalapeño pepper (1)

Poblano pepper (1)

Tomatillos (4)

Fresh cilantro

Limes (wedges for serving, optional)

Salmon fillets (1 pound; Pacific wild-caught preferred)

Jane's Krazy Mixed-Up Salt

Canola oil cooking spray

Yellow squash and zucchini (suggested side)

cilantro-lime rice

Total time: 5 minutes

Lunch Leftovers

This is a super simple way to jazz up leftover rice or microwave-ready rice.

2 cups precooked brown rice or microwaveable whole-grain

1 teaspoon lime zest

4 teaspoons lime juice

1½ tablespoons chopped fresh cilantro

½ teaspoon salt

Cracked black pepper, to taste

GROCERY LIST:
Limes (2 needed for juice and zest)

Fresh cilantro

Cooked brown rice or microwaveable wholegrain rice (2 cups)

Salt

Cracked black pepper

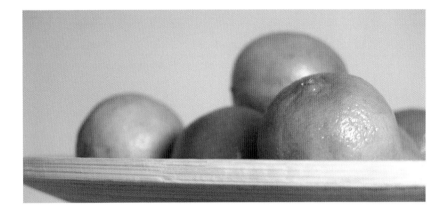

1. Place rice in a microwave-safe bowl and microwave until warm. Stir at 30–60 second intervals.

2. Once rice is warm, stir in remaining ingredients and enjoy.

Yield: 6 servings
(serving size: ⅓ cup)

Nutrient Breakdown:
Calories 70

Fat 0.5g

Cholesterol 0mg

Sodium 200mg

Carbohydrate 15g

Fiber 1g

Protein 2g

Plate Plan choices:
1 starch

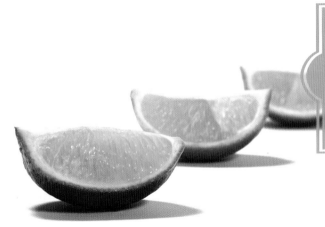

WE LOVE LIMES! We are highlighting them this week, so go ahead and buy a few!

- super flavorful
- packed with vitamin C
- add a light, fresh flavor to foods

steakhouse chicken

The marinade and grill seasoning create a rich, steak-like flavor for chicken. We suggest doubling this recipe for use in the next few days, or cutting it into strips to freeze for use anytime.

Lunch Leftovers

Hands-on time: 18 minutes   Total time: 50 minutes (includes 30-minute marinating time)

Basic Steak Marinade
2 tablespoons extra-virgin olive oil

1 tablespoon Worcestershire sauce

2 tablespoons reduced-sodium soy sauce

2 garlic cloves, minced

1 tablespoon lime juice

Chicken
1 pound boneless, skinless chicken breasts

1½ teaspoons grill seasoning of choice

Canola oil (for oiling the grill grates)

GROCERY LIST:

Garlic cloves (2)

Lime juice (1 tablespoon)

Boneless, skinless chicken breasts (1 pound)

Worcestershire sauce

Reduced-sodium soy sauce

Grill seasoning of choice

Extra-virgin olive oil

Canola oil (to oil grill grates)

1. Combine marinade ingredients (olive oil through lime juice) in a small bowl and set aside.

2. Place the chicken in a gallon-sized plastic zip-top bag (leave the bag unsealed but fold over the open end). Pound the thick end of the chicken thin with the flat side of a meat-mallet to create uniform thickness. Pour the marinade into the bag and seal. Place the bag in a shallow bowl or plate and marinate in the refrigerator for 30 minutes or more.

3. Oil clean grill grates with a folded paper towel soaked in canola oil.

4. When ready to grill, preheat the grill to medium-high heat (350–400°F). Remove chicken to a clean plate, discard marinade, and sprinkle grill seasoning over the chicken.

5. Grill chicken on one side for 4 minutes undisturbed. Flip and cook on the second side 4 minutes or until done (chicken is done when the internal temperature registers 165°F on a meat thermometer).

Yield: 4 servings
(serving size: 3 ounces)

Nutrient Breakdown:
Calories 150

Fat 4.5g (1g saturated fat)

Cholesterol 75mg

Sodium 350mg

Carbohydrate 0g

Fiber 0mg

Protein 24g

Plate Plan choices:
3 very lean meats

I used to wait until my husband got home to do the grilling, but one day I thought, "Hey now, this girl can work a gas grill! I'm getting this weeknight fill-the-grill dinner going!" And "fill the grill" I do! I typically grill more meat than I need for the current meal to freeze in strips for another busy night, and I always fill my grill basket with veggies... grape tomatoes, whole mini peppers and onion wedges are my go-to combo: minimal prep required. If there's any room left, I add a few cobs of corn, husk and all. Week 6 has a fill-the-grill weekend you will love!

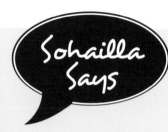

Sohailla Says

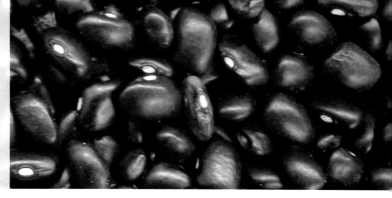

 COUNTDOWN QUICKER-FIX:

To speed up this quick recipe, use frozen chopped onions and peppers, or drop your peppers, onion and garlic cloves into a food processor. Also, if you have preportioned frozen beans that you've cooked in the slow cooker as directed at the start of the Countdown, this is a great time to use those.

cuban-style black beans

Quicker-Fix   Lunch Leftovers

These are sure to become a family favorite!

Hands-on time: 7 minutes
Total time: 17 minutes

1½ tablespoons extra-virgin olive oil

1 small onion, chopped (about 1 cup)

½ green bell pepper, finely chopped (about ½ cup)

½ red bell pepper, finely chopped (about ½ cup)

3 garlic cloves, minced

¼ teaspoon salt

½ teaspoon dried oregano

½ teaspoon cumin

2 14.5-ounce cans no-salt-added black beans

1 lime, divided use

Fresh cilantro (optional, but delicious)

Chopped onion (optional, but delicious)

1. Place a large nonstick skillet over medium heat and add oil. Once the oil is hot, add the onion and peppers. Sauté over medium heat for 5 minutes, stirring occasionally.

2. Add the garlic, salt, oregano, cumin and one can of beans with the bean liquid.* Drain and rinse the other can of beans and add to the skillet. Allow mixture to cook for an additional 5 minutes.

3. Cut the lime in half and squeeze the juice from one half into the beans just before serving. Serve with remaining lime cut into wedges and optional garnishes if desired. (Freeze any extras in 1½-cup portions to use in the Vegetarian Chili on Day 25.)

Yield: 8 servings
(serving size: ½ cup)

Nutrient Breakdown:
Calories 90

Fat 2.5g (0g saturated fat)

Cholesterol 0mg

Sodium 280mg

Carbohydrate 17g

Fiber 6g

Protein 5g

Plate Plan choices:
1 starch, ½ vegetable

GROCERY LIST:

Lime (1)

Onion (1 plus additional for garnish if desired)

Green bell pepper (½ pepper)

Red bell pepper (½ pepper)

Garlic cloves (3)

Fresh cilantro (optional)

Reduced-sodium black beans (2 14.5-ounce cans)

Salt

Dried oregano

Cumin

Extra-virgin olive oil

*Using the liquid from one can of beans helps to thicken the soup, and draining the other can keeps the sodium level in check.

roasted asparagus with garlic and lemon

Lunch Leftovers

Club Favorite

This is a pretty quick recipe, but to speed it up even more, simply roast asparagus with salt, pepper, and oil and serve with lemon wedges. If you plan to serve tonight's entire meal as leftovers, you'll want to double this recipe.

Hands-on time: 15 minutes   Total time: 25 minutes

Canola oil cooking spray

1 bunch asparagus (about 1 pound), trimmed

2 teaspoons extra-virgin olive oil

$\frac{1}{8}$ teaspoon black pepper

$\frac{1}{8}$ teaspoon salt

Zest of half a lemon

1 tablespoon lemon juice

2 cloves garlic, minced

2 tablespoons pine nuts

GROCERY LIST:
Fresh asparagus (1 bunch is about 1 pound)

Garlic cloves (2)

Lemon (1 tablespoon juice and zest)

Pine nuts (2 tablespoons)

Black pepper

Salt

Extra-virgin olive oil

Canola oil cooking spray

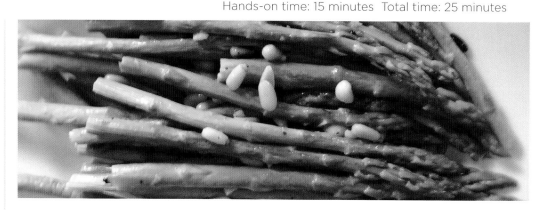

1. Preheat the oven to 400°F. Line a baking pan with aluminum foil (for easy clean up) and coat with cooking spray. Lay asparagus on the baking pan in a single layer.

2. Combine the next 6 ingredients (oil through garlic) and whisk together. Drizzle the mixture over asparagus and toss to coat.

3. Roast for 8–10 minutes, turning halfway through cooking time.

4. While asparagus cooks, toast the pine nuts in a small, dry nonstick skillet over medium heat. (You may be tempted to skip the toasting step, but the flavor is worth the effort). Toast the nuts for 1–2 minutes, stirring or shaking the pan frequently to avoid burning. As the nuts become fragrant and begin to change color, remove them from the heat. You will want to stay close as these are expensive and will burn easily.

5. Transfer asparagus to a serving platter and sprinkle with toasted pine nuts.

Yield: 4 servings
(serving size: about ½ cup)

Nutrient Breakdown:
Calories 70

Fat 4g (0.5g saturated fat)

Cholesterol 0mg

Sodium 90mg

Carbohydrate 7g

Fiber 4g

Protein 2g

Plate Plan choices:
1 vegetable, 1 fat

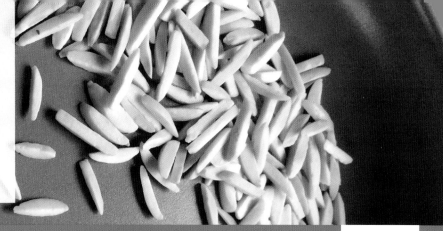

COUNTDOWN QUICKER-FIX:

Countdown Quicker-Fix: To save a few minutes of both cooking time and cleaning time, simply steam the green beans and toss with oil. Add almonds and seasoning salt afterwards, using garlic powder instead of minced garlic.

DAY 36

pair with Planned-Over Best Ever Spinach Lasagna

Easy Meal

green beans with toasted almonds

Quicker-Fix

Nuts add that important crunch factor we all love, not to mention healthy fat, fiber, nutrients, and of course, flavor.

Hands-on time: 7 minutes

1 12-ounce microwavable package fresh green beans

½ tablespoons extra-virgin olive oil

2 garlic cloves, minced

2 tablespoons chopped toasted almonds (or nut of choice)

½ teaspoons Jane's Krazy Mixed-Up Salt

GROCERY LIST:
Fresh green beans (12-ounce package)

Garlic cloves (2)

Toasted almonds

Jane's Krazy Mixed-Up Salt

Extra-virgin olive oil

1. Steam green beans (as directed on their package or in a microwave-safe bowl). To steam green beans in a bowl, place clean, trimmed green beans in a microwave-safe bowl, add ¼ cup water, and cover with a damp paper towel. Microwave for 2–4 minutes (depending on how tender you like your green beans).

2. Add oil to a large nonstick skillet and place over medium-high heat. Once the oil is hot, add the garlic and cook for 30 seconds. Add the drained green beans and salt, stirring to combine.

3. Transfer beans to a serving dish and top with toasted almonds.

Yield: 4 servings
(serving size: 1 cup)

Nutrient Breakdown:
Calories 60

Fat 3.5g

Cholesterol 0mg

Sodium 150mg

Carbohydrate 7g

Fiber 3g

Protein 2g

Plate Plan choices:
2 vegetables, ½ fat

Because green beans are a staple vegetable in most homes, we've given you three simple variations of preparation methods for them. Check out Day 48 and Day 21 for alternate options.

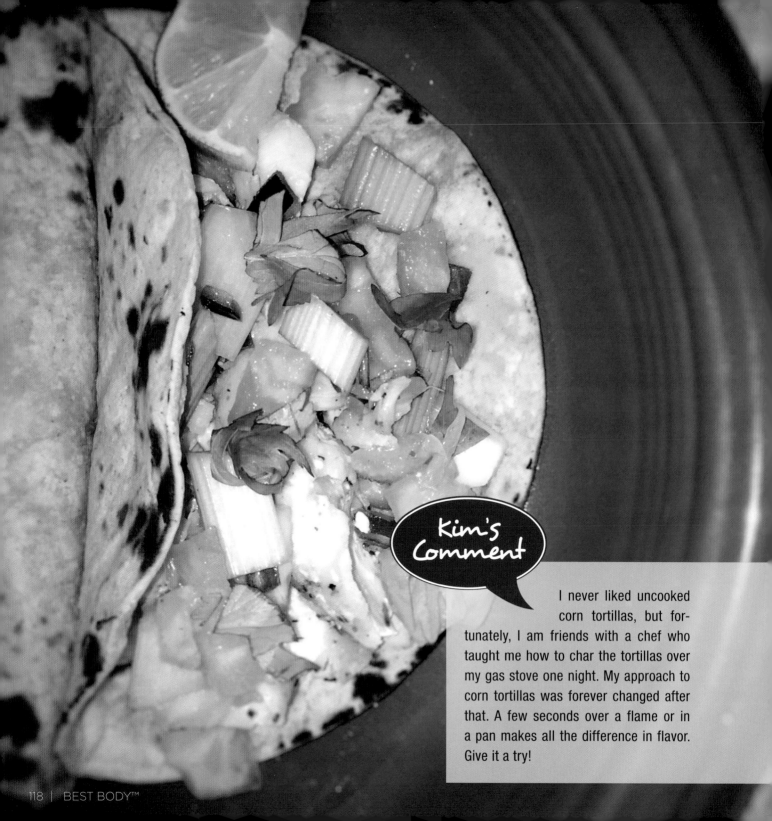

Kim's Comment

I never liked uncooked corn tortillas, but fortunately, I am friends with a chef who taught me how to char the tortillas over my gas stove one night. My approach to corn tortillas was forever changed after that. A few seconds over a flame or in a pan makes all the difference in flavor. Give it a try!

Easy Meal

jerk fish tacos with pineapple salsa

Total time: 20 minutes

Club Favorite

This is one of the most delicious ways to get some omega-3s!

suggested side:
steamed broccoli

4 4–5-ounce fresh or frozen cod fillets or other mild white fish (soak or thaw in milk, if desired)

½ cup diced pineapple (canned in juice, frozen or fresh are all acceptable forms)

¼ cup chopped celery

2 tablespoons chopped red onion

¼ teaspoon chopped jalapeño

1 tablespoon chopped fresh cilantro

Lime juice (1 tablespoon)

4 teaspoons Jerk seasoning

1 tablespoon canola oil, divided

8 corn tortillas

Finely chopped lettuce

1. Before cooking, pat fish dry with paper towels. While preparing the salsa, allow the fish to rest on paper towels to soak up any remaining moisture (the more liquid soaked up in this step the better, as it will allow the fish to cook faster and soak up flavors).

2. In a medium bowl, combine the salsa ingredients and set aside or refrigerate until needed.

3. Place a nonstick skillet over medium heat and add ½ tablespoon of oil. As the skillet heats up, season the fish on both sides with Jerk seasoning. Once the oil is hot, add half the fish and cook 2 minutes on the first side, flip, and cook 1–2 additional minutes or until done (fish is done when it is opaque throughout). Repeat with the remaining oil and fish. Wipe the pan out to cook the tortillas.

4. To heat the tortillas, place the dry skillet over medium-high heat and add the tortillas in a single layer. Cook them for about 30–60 seconds on each side, allowing them to char just a little (if you heat them this way, they will be more flavorful and will remain pliable enough to form tacos). If you have a gas stove, you could also char them directly over the gas flames, turning them with tongs. The direct flame method will take less time but requires more attention to avoid burning the tortillas. Keep tortillas warm by covering with a clean damp towel.

5. To serve, fill the tacos with equal portions of fish and top with salsa and lettuce.

Yield: 4 servings
(serving size: 2 tacos, 3 tablespoons salsa, and lettuce)

Nutrient Breakdown:
Calories 300

Fat 6g (300mg omega-3 fatty acids)

Cholesterol 50mg

Sodium 460mg

Carbohydrate 32g

Fiber 4g

Protein 29g

Plate Plan choices:
2 starches, 4 lean meats

GROCERY LIST:

Pineapple (½ cup diced, canned in juice, frozen or fresh are acceptable)

Celery

Red onion

Jalapeño

Finely chopped romaine lettuce (or other crunchy lettuce)

Fresh cilantro

Lime juice (1 tablespoon)

Corn tortillas (8)

Jerk seasoning

Fresh or frozen cod, or other mild white fish (4 4–5 ounce fillets)

Canola oil

Brocolli (suggested side)

"These are great! I will be making them again and again. The sweet pineapple is a nice balance to the spice."

—BECKY, 57

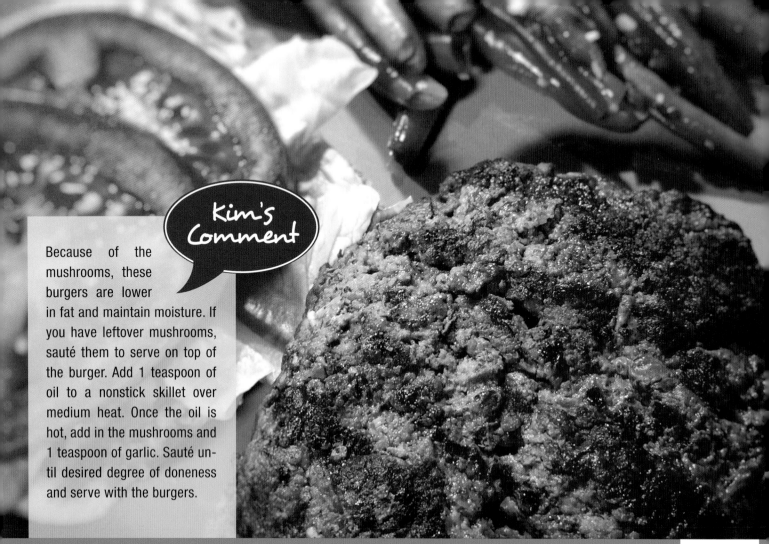

Kim's Comment

Because of the mushrooms, these burgers are lower in fat and maintain moisture. If you have leftover mushrooms, sauté them to serve on top of the burger. Add 1 teaspoon of oil to a nonstick skillet over medium heat. Once the oil is hot, add in the mushrooms and 1 teaspoon of garlic. Sauté until desired degree of doneness and serve with the burgers.

DAY 34

Easy Meal

all-american backyard burger

Mushrooms and mayonnaise keep this lean meat moist. Searing the meat first also helps to develop a nice flavor and produce good color.

suggested side: Refreshing Rainbow Salad
(see Pre-Countdown Day recipe and grocery list)

Total time: 22 minutes

½ cup finely chopped mushrooms (see Kim's Comment)

1½ teaspoons salt-free garlic and herb seasoning (such as Mrs. Dash)

1 teaspoon reduced-sodium soy sauce

1 tablespoon canola mayonnaise

1 pound ground sirloin or lean ground beef (90% lean or more)

¼ teaspoon salt

4 whole-wheat buns or sandwich thins

4 slices lettuce

4 slices tomato

1. Combine first 4 ingredients (mushrooms through mayonnaise) in a medium-sized bowl. Add the ground beef and mix gently to combine, taking care not to overmix.

2. Divide meat into 4 equal portions and make into patties. Sprinkle salt over the burger patties.

3. Oil clean grill grates with a folded paper towel soaked in canola oil. Preheat one side of the grill to high heat and the other side to medium-low heat.

4. Cook the burgers over high heat for 3–4 minutes on each side (this will sear the meat). Finish cooking the burgers over medium-low heat with the lid down until done, about 6–8 minutes depending on the thickness of the burger (burgers are done when the internal temperature reaches 160°F on a meat thermometer).

5. Serve the burgers on buns with lettuce, tomato, and condiments of choice.

Yield: 4 servings
(serving size: 1 burger with bun)

Nutrient Breakdown:
Calories 270

Fat 8g (2.5g saturated fat)

Cholesterol 60mg

Sodium 470mg

Carbohydrate 24g

Fiber 4g

Protein 27g

Plate Plan choices:
1½ starches, 3½ lean meats, 1 vegetable (with lettuce and tomato)

GROCERY LIST:

Mushrooms

Lettuce

Tomato (1)

Ground sirloin or lean ground beef (1 pound)

Whole-wheat buns or sandwich thins (4)

Reduced-sodium soy sauce

Canola mayonnaise

Salt-free garlic and herb seasoning (such as Mrs. Dash)

Salt

Refreshing Rainbow Salad (suggested side)

TO PAN FRY:

Put 1 teaspoon canola oil in a nonstick skillet and place over medium-high heat. When the oil is hot, swirl the oil in the pan to coat and add the hamburgers. Cook the burgers 3 minutes, flip, and cook 3 additional minutes. Reduce heat to medium. Add 1–2 tablespoons water and cover pan with a lid. Cook for 2 more minutes or until 160°F internal temperature is reached.

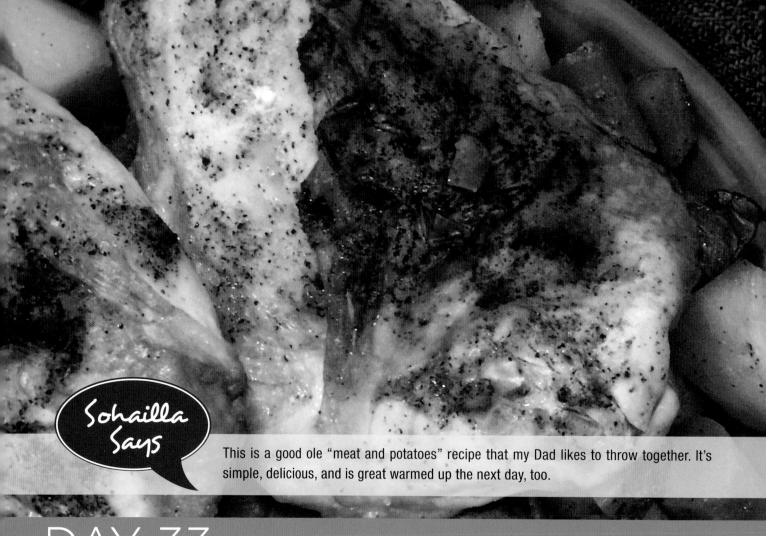

Sohailla Says

This is a good ole "meat and potatoes" recipe that my Dad likes to throw together. It's simple, delicious, and is great warmed up the next day, too.

DAY 33

dad's oven-roasted chicken with vegetables

Lunch Leftovers

This is Sohailla's Dad's recipe with a few tweaks by Kim. It is a great basic recipe! Feel free to add other seasonings and herbs.

suggested side: steamed brocolli *(and whole-grain rolls, if desired)*

Hands-on time: 26 minutes
Total time: 1 hour 26 minutes

2 tablespoons extra-virgin olive oil

2 tablespoons salt-free seasoning (such as Mrs. Dash), divided

3 garlic cloves, minced

8–10 small red potatoes, quartered or further cut if on the larger side (about 1 pound)

2 pounds baby carrots or peeled whole carrots (cut into 1-inch pieces with thick pieces halved, or quartered if especially large)

2 medium onions, sliced

3–4 pounds of split chicken breasts* (about 4)

½ teaspoon salt

Paprika

GROCERY LIST:

Red potatoes, small (1 pound)

Baby carrots or peeled whole carrots (2 pounds)

Onions (2 medium)

Garlic cloves (3)

Split chicken breasts (3–4 pounds)

Salt-free seasoning (such as Mrs. Dash)

Salt

Paprika

Extra-virgin olive oil

Whole-grain rolls (suggested side, if desired)

Salad fixings (suggested side)

1. Preheat the oven to 400°F.

2. Cover a large roasting pan (or 9x13-inch pan) with aluminum foil. Pour oil and 1½ tablespoons seasoning over the foil, add garlic and vegetables and toss to coat in oil. Place the chicken pieces on top of the vegetables.

3. In a small bowl, mix the remaining ½ tablespoon seasoning with the salt. Using your fingers, gently separate the skin from the chicken and work the seasoning under the skin into the meat. Sprinkle paprika over the chicken until covered.

4. Place the pan on the middle rack of the oven and bake for 45–60 minutes or until done (chicken is done when an internal temperature of 165°F is reached on a meat thermometer). Check the temperature at 45 minutes, with the goal of cooking the chicken completely without overcooking.

Yield: 8 servings
(serving size: ½ chicken breast and 1 cup vegetables)

Nutrient Breakdown:
Calories 340

Fat 10g (2.5g saturated fat)

Cholesterol 120mg

Sodium 430mg

Carbohydrate 25g

Fiber 4g

Protein 41g

Plate Plan choices:
3 vegetables, 1 starch, 5 very lean meats, 1 fat

Kim's Comment

I just love a Sunday roast. It brings back such great memories of walking into my Granny's house after church and smelling a delicious meal… usually including roasted meat of some kind. You may notice a few of our weeks include a roast on the weekend; we do this to set you up with leftovers to use during the week.

*Cooking the chicken with the skin on will help keep it from drying out, but please do remove it before eating. We are all for flavor but with a bit less saturated fat when possible.

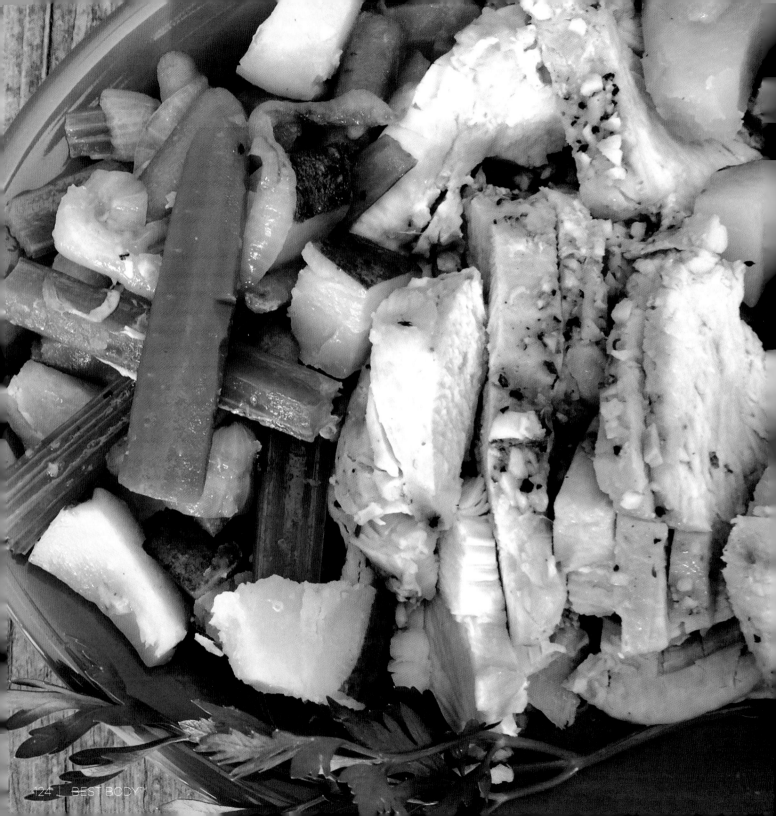

recipes & menu:
week four

> " Make [food] simple and let things taste of what they are."
>
> — CURNONSKY, FRENCH WRITER

menu key:

Slow-Cooker

Club Favorite

Easy Meal

Lunch Leftovers

Pricey Meal

Quicker-Fix

DAY 32
Hearty Black Bean Soup
Suggested side: raw veggie sticks

DAY 31
Pistachio-Crusted Tilapia
Barley with Spinach and Corn
Suggested side: steamed beets

DAY 30
Mediterranean Chicken Over Orzo
Suggested side: crackers with hummus appetizer

DAY 29
Slow-Cooked Pineapple Pork
Sautéed Sugar Snap Peas
Suggested side: brown rice

DAY 28
Broiled Salmon
Super-Food Salad with Perfect Dressing
Pita Chips

DAY 27
Grilled Steak with Garlic and Lime
Roasted or Grilled Cabbage
Edamame Pasta Salad

DAY 26
One-Dish Roasted Turkey Dinner
Suggested side: green salad

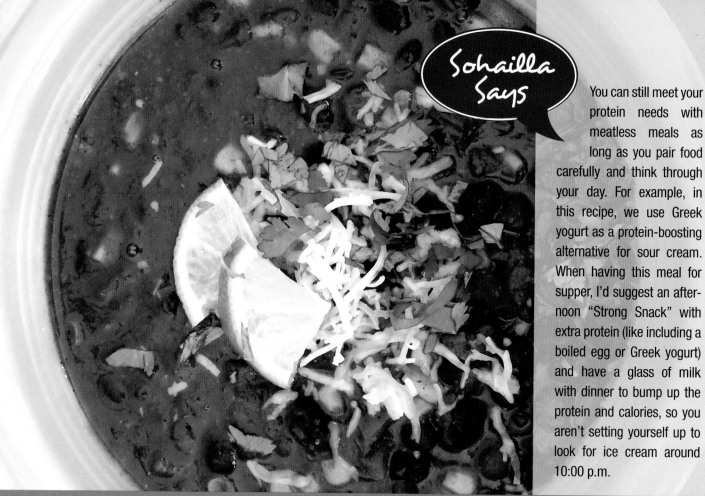

DAY 32

hearty black bean soup

Total time: 25 minutes

 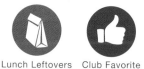

Lunch Leftovers   Club Favorite

This hearty Best Body Club favorite can be made spicy or mild depending on the heat of the diced tomatoes. This is a fall and winter staple at Sohailla's house; it's perfect for lunch the next day, too.

suggested side: raw veggie sticks

1 tablespoon extra-virgin olive oil

1 green bell pepper, diced
(about 1 cup)

1 medium onion, chopped
(about 1½ cups)

2 cloves garlic, minced

2 10-ounce cans diced tomatoes
with chilies

4 14.5-ounce cans black beans,
drained and rinsed (equal to 1 pound
cooked black beans or 6 cups)

1 cup frozen corn

4 cups of unsalted vegetable broth

2 tablespoons chili powder

2 teaspoons ground cumin

1 teaspoon Jane's Krazy
Mixed-Up Salt

Toppings
¾ cup reduced-fat shredded cheese

¾ cup plain nonfat Greek yogurt

Chopped fresh cilantro (optional)

Lime wedges (optional)

1. Add oil to a large pot or Dutch oven and place over medium heat. Once the oil is hot, add the pepper, onion, and garlic. Sauté for 3–4 minutes until the vegetables begin to soften. Add the remaining 7 ingredients (tomatoes through salt) to the pot and mix well.

2. Scoop out 3 cups of the soup before it heats, and puree it in a blender until smooth (this will thicken the soup nicely). Return the puree to the pot and stir to combine. Bring the soup to a boil, reduce the heat and simmer for about 10 minutes, allowing the soup to thicken.

3. Serve with 2 tablespoons each of cheese and Greek yogurt.

Yield: 6 servings
(serving size: 1½ cups and 2 tablespoons each of cheese and Greek yogurt)

Nutrient Breakdown:
Calories 250

Fat 2g (1g saturated fat)

Cholesterol 5mg

Sodium 486mg

Carbohydrate 50g

Fiber 15g

Protein 18g

Plate Plan choices:
2½ starches,
2 vegetables,
2 lean meats

"The recipe is easy to make for a quick meal on a cool evening, with plenty to take to work for lunch the next day."
—SUZANNE, 48

GROCERY LIST:

Green bell pepper (1)	Fresh cilantro (optional, but delicious)	Diced tomatoes with chilies such as RoTel (2 10-ounce cans)	Plain, nonfat Greek yogurt
Onion (1)			Frozen corn
Garlic cloves (2)	No-salt-added black beans (4 14.5-ounce cans or 6 cups precooked)	Unsalted vegetable broth	Chili powder
Lime (wedges for serving, optional)		Reduced-fat shredded cheese	Ground cumin
			Jane's Krazy Mixed-Up Salt
			Extra-virgin olive oil

Easy Meal

pistachio-crusted tilapia

Hands-on time: 7 minutes
Total time: 20 minutes

The pistachios make a nice crunchy coating for this delicate white fish. Gourmet goodness!

suggested side: steamed beets

Canola oil cooking spray

4 4-ounce fresh or frozen tilapia fillets (soak or thaw in milk, if desired)

1 teaspoon Jane's Krazy Mixed-Up Salt

2 tablespoons unseasoned breadcrumbs

3 tablespoons finely chopped pistachios (pecans or walnuts work, too)

2 teaspoons extra-virgin olive oil

Lemon wedges (optional)

GROCERY LIST:

Tilapia (4 4-ounce fillets)

Unseasoned breadcrumbs

Pistachios

Jane's Krazy Mixed-Up Salt

Extra-virgin olive oil

Canola oil cooking spray

Lemon (wedges for serving, optional)

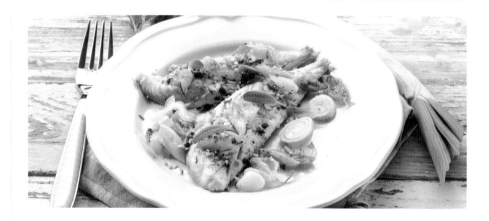

1. Preheat the oven to 350°F. Spray an 8x8-inch baking pan with cooking spray.

2. Pat fish dry with paper towels. While gathering ingredients allow the fish to rest on paper towels to soak up any remaining moisture (the more liquid soaked up in this step the better; this allows the coating to adhere and flavor the fish during cooking).

3. Place fish in prepared baking dish and sprinkle evenly with seasoning salt. In a small bowl, combine breadcrumbs and pistachios. Top fish with the breadcrumb mixture, pressing it into the fish gently with your fingers, and drizzle with oil. Bake for 12–14 minutes or until done. Serve with a squeeze of lemon if desired.

Yield: 4 servings
(serving size: 1 fillet)

Nutrient Breakdown:
Calories 180

Fat 7g
(1.5g saturated fat)

Cholesterol 55mg

Sodium 330mg

Carbohydrate 4g

Fiber 1g

Protein 25g

Plate Plan choices:
3 very lean meats,
1 fat

barley with spinach and corn

Total time: 20 minutes

Lunch Leftovers

This is a wonderful side dish and a great way to use up any precooked barley or rice in your fridge or freezer: the perfect chance to transform leftovers into something brand new.

Canola oil cooking spray

1½ teaspoons extra-virgin olive oil

½ cup chopped onion

2 cloves garlic, minced

1 cup frozen corn, thawed

½ teaspoon salt

¼ teaspoon dried thyme or 1 teaspoon fresh thyme

6 cups roughly chopped fresh spinach (5 ounces)

2 cups precooked barley (or brown rice)

2 tablespoons grated Parmesan cheese

GROCERY LIST:

Fresh spinach (5 ounces or 6 cups)

Onion (1)

Garlic cloves (2)

Frozen corn (1 cup)

Grated Parmesan cheese

Barley or brown rice
(1 cup uncooked or 2 cups cooked)

Salt

Dried thyme leaves

Extra-virgin olive oil

Canola oil cooking spray

1. Coat a nonstick skillet with cooking spray and add oil. Place skillet over medium heat.

2. Once the oil is hot, add the onion, garlic, corn, salt and thyme, sauté for 2–3 minutes until onion is soft and thyme is aromatic.

3. Add chopped spinach and barley, stirring until the spinach is wilted (about 2–3 minutes).

4. Top with Parmesan cheese to serve.

Yield: 6 servings
(serving size: ½ cup barley and 1 teaspoon Parmesan cheese)

Nutrient Breakdown:
Calories 110

Fat 2.5g
(0.5g saturated fat, 1g monounsaturated fat)

Cholesterol 0mg

Sodium 260mg

Carbohydrate 23g

Fiber 4g

Protein 3g

Plate Plan choices:
1 starch, 1 vegetable

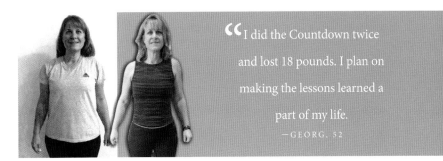

"I did the Countdown twice and lost 18 pounds. I plan on making the lessons learned a part of my life.
—GEORG, 52

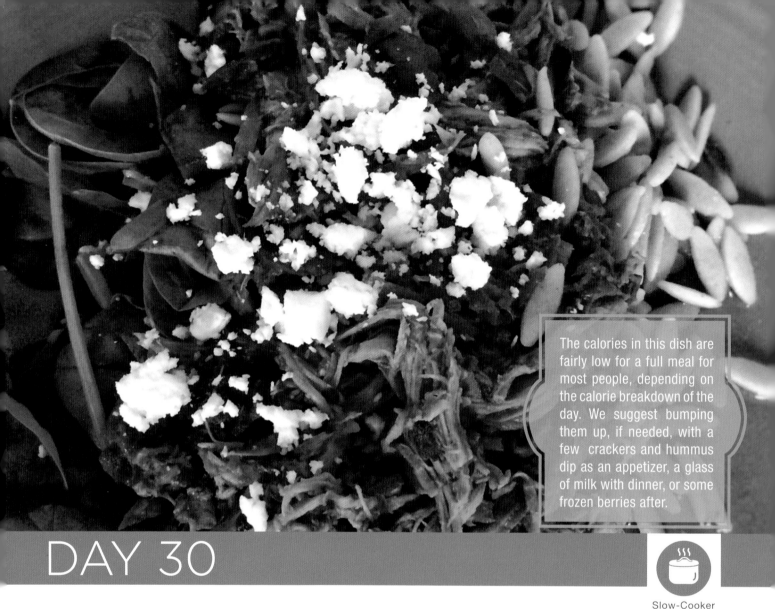

The calories in this dish are fairly low for a full meal for most people, depending on the calorie breakdown of the day. We suggest bumping them up, if needed, with a few crackers and hummus dip as an appetizer, a glass of milk with dinner, or some frozen berries after.

DAY 30

Slow-Cooker

mediterranean chicken over orzo

Lunch Leftovers

The sun-dried tomatoes and olives are key flavor enhancers in this dish. The eggplant melts beautifully into the chicken and provides a nice creamy texture. However, if eggplant is not available, zucchini or squash make a suitable substitution.

suggested side: crackers or raw veggies with hummus

Hands-on time: 20 minutes
Total time: 8 hours and 20 minutes
(includes slow-cooker time)

1½ pounds boneless, skinless chicken breasts

½ teaspoon Jane's Krazy Mixed-Up Salt

¼ teaspoon black pepper

1 cup unsalted chicken broth

½ cup sliced sun-dried tomatoes

4 ounces sliced mushrooms

1 6-ounce jar marinated artichoke hearts, drained and chopped

1 small (or ½ medium) eggplant chopped into ½-inch pieces

5 garlic cloves, thinly sliced

3 cups cooked whole-wheat orzo (or whole-grain of choice)

¼–½ cup Kalamata olives, pitted and sliced

6 tablespoons crumbled feta cheese (1½ ounces)

GROCERY LIST:
Eggplant (1 small or ½ medium)

Garlic cloves (5)

Boneless, skinless chicken breasts (1½ pounds)

Whole-wheat orzo or grain of choice

Unsalted chicken broth

Sun-dried tomatoes (½ cup)

Sliced mushrooms (4 ounces)

Marinated artichoke hearts (6-ounce jar)

Kalamata olives (¼–½ cup)

Feta cheese

Jane's Krazy Mixed-Up Salt

Black pepper

Whole-grain rolls (suggested side, if desired)

Salad fixings (suggested side)

1. Season the chicken breasts with seasoning salt and pepper and place in a large slow cooker.
2. Add the next 6 ingredients (broth through garlic) to the slow cooker. Cook on low for 8 hours (or on high for 4–6 hours).
3. When the chicken is done, remove the chicken and shred it (it may fall apart). Mix shredded chicken into the vegetables. Serve over orzo and top with olives and feta cheese.

Yield: 6 servings
(serving size: 1 cup chicken mixture and ½ cup orzo)

Nutrient Breakdown:
Calories 320

Fat 7g (1.5g saturated fat, 1g monounsaturated fat)

Cholesterol 75mg

Sodium 470mg

Carbohydrate 33g

Fiber 7g

Protein 33g

Plate Plan choices:
1½ starches, 4 lean meats, 3 vegetables

Kim's Comment

For a veggie boost with the Mediterranean Chicken recipe, serve with our Simple Sautéed Spinach or toss a handful of raw spinach on top of the orzo and serve the chicken over the spinach. The heat from the chicken will gently wilt the spinach.

Easy Meal   Slow-Cooker

slow-cooked pineapple pork

Hands-on time: 6 minutes
Total time: 8 hours and 6 minutes
(includes time in the slow cooker)

Lunch Leftovers

This recipe has the perfect balance of savory and subtle sweetness to satisfy any appetite.

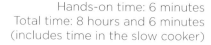

suggested side: brown rice

2 pounds pork loin (thick chops, or use loin or loin roast cut into chops)

1 teaspoon Jane's Krazy Mixed-Up Salt

½ teaspoon Greek seasoning (such as Cavender's)

½ large green bell pepper cut into strips (or frozen mixed peppers)

1 20-ounce can pineapple chunks in juice

1 tablespoon reduced-sodium teriyaki sauce

1–2 green onions, chopped (optional garnish)

GROCERY LIST:
Green pepper (1 pepper or frozen mixed peppers)

Green onion (optional garnish)

Pork loin thick chops (2 pounds)

Pineapple chunks in juice (1 20-ounce can)

Reduced-sodium teriyaki sauce

Jane's Krazy Mixed-Up Salt

Cavender's Greek seasoning

Brown rice (suggested side)

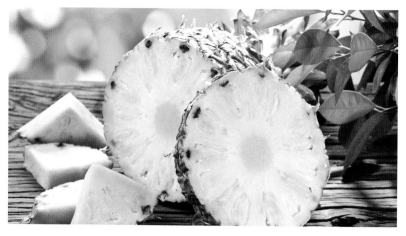

1. Trim excess fat from pork (there should not be much).

2. Place the pork in the slow cooker and sprinkle with seasonings. Add green pepper strips, the pineapple (with juice) and teriyaki sauce to the slow cooker. Cover and cook on low for 8–10 hours.

Yield: 8 servings
(serving size: about 1½ cups)

Nutrient Breakdown:
Calories 190

Fat 7g (saturated fat 1.5g)

Cholesterol 60mg

Sodium 260mg

Carbohydrate 13g

Protein 19g

Plate Plan choices:
1 fruit, 3 lean meats

COUNTDOWN QUICKER-FIX:

Use either fresh or frozen sugar snap peas in the steamer bags. Season them after they are cooked but still warm. For example, carefully cut the steamer bag open, add chopped green onions, garlic, salt and pepper to the bag, re-close the bag with a clip, shake, and let sit for about 30–60 seconds, which allows the steam to mellow the raw onion and garlic.

sautéed sugar snap peas

Hands-on time: 5 minutes
Total time: 10 minutes

Quicker-Fix

Snap peas are crisp, sweet, and succulent, making them one of the easiest vegetables to convince Kim's kids to eat. They can be "snapped" into pieces and mixed into salads, or eaten whole as an appetizer, snack, or side dish.

Canola oil cooking spray

½ teaspoon extra-virgin olive oil

1 garlic clove, minced

2 green onions, chopped

1 8-ounce package sugar snap peas, washed and strings removed

⅛ teaspoon salt

Cracked black pepper, to taste

GROCERY LIST:
Garlic clove (1)

Green onions (2)

Sugar snap peas (8 ounces)

Extra-virgin olive oil

Salt

Cracked black pepper

Canola oil cooking spray

1. Spray a large nonstick skillet with cooking spray, add oil, and place over medium-high heat. When the oil is hot, add the onions and garlic. Sauté for 30 seconds.

2. Add the snap peas and cook for 2 minutes, shaking the pan to flip-stir the peas (or simply stir the peas). They should be warm throughout but still bright green and crisp. Sprinkle with salt and pepper to taste.

Yield: 4 servings *(serving size: ¾ cup)*

Nutrient Breakdown:
Calories 35

Fat 1g

Cholesterol 0mg

Sodium 75mg

Carbohydrate 7g

Fiber 1g

Protein 1g

Plate Plan choices: 1½ vegetables

Kim's Comment

I may have just coined the term "flip-stir!" This term describes a feeling and a cooking move all in one. You "flip-stir" when you feel confident and a touch feisty, and therefore you believe you can flip the food in the pan. This facilitates even cooking, eliminating the need to stir. I feel this way when cooking these peas. I wish you the same level of confidence in the kitchen as well. Happy "flip-stirring" to you!

VARIATIONS:

Lemon-Mint: Sprinkle with 1 teaspoon chopped mint, ½ teaspoon lemon zest and 1 teaspoon lemon juice.

Sesame-Soy: Omit salt and add 2 teaspoons reduced-sodium soy sauce to pan during cooking. Once done, sprinkle the snap peas with 1 teaspoon sesame seeds. (117mg sodium)

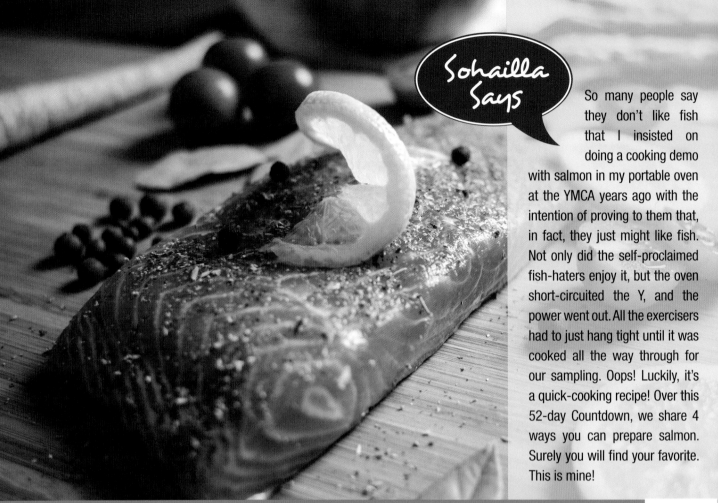

Sohailla Says

So many people say they don't like fish that I insisted on doing a cooking demo with salmon in my portable oven at the YMCA years ago with the intention of proving to them that, in fact, they just might like fish. Not only did the self-proclaimed fish-haters enjoy it, but the oven short-circuited the Y, and the power went out. All the exercisers had to just hang tight until it was cooked all the way through for our sampling. Oops! Luckily, it's a quick-cooking recipe! Over this 52-day Countdown, we share 4 ways you can prepare salmon. Surely you will find your favorite. This is mine!

DAY 28

Pricey Meal

broiled salmon

Total time: 20 minutes

Lunch Leftovers

Club Favorite

Salmon is a wonderfully flavorful fish. The lemon juice and seasoning mix add a bright flavor while keeping the recipe super simple.

¼ cup lemon juice

2 teaspoons extra-virgin olive oil

1 tablespoon salt-free garlic and herb seasoning (such as Mrs. Dash)

¼ teaspoon Greek seasoning (such as Cavender's)

Fresh or dried dill, as desired

4 4-ounce salmon fillets, Pacific wild-caught preferred (soak or thaw in milk, if desired)

GROCERY LIST:
Lemon juice (¼ cup)

Fresh or dried dill (optional)

Salmon (1 pound, Pacific wild-caught preferred)

Salt-free garlic and herb seasoning (such as Mrs. Dash)

Greek seasoning (such as Cavender's)

Extra-virgin olive oil

1. Preheat the broiler. Mix lemon juice, oil, and seasonings together.

2. Pat the fish dry with paper towels. While gathering ingredients, allow the fish to rest on paper towels to soak up any remaining liquid (the more liquid soaked up in this step the better, as it allows the seasoning to adhere and flavor the fish during cooking).

3. Drizzle the seasoning mix over a shallow foil-covered baking dish or pan. Dredge salmon through the seasoning mix on both sides until covered. Sprinkle with dill if desired.

4. Broil for 4–7 minutes on each side, depending on the thickness of the fish. When turning the salmon, remove the skin easily by sliding a spatula under the skin. Add more dill, if desired.

Yield: 4 servings
(serving size: 1 fillet)

Nutrient Breakdown:
Calories 189

Fat 7g (1g saturated fat, 1200mg omega-3 fatty acids)

Sodium 459mg

Carbohydrate 2g

Fiber 0g

Protein 23g

Plate Plan choices:
3 lean meats

When turning the salmon, add grape tomatoes to roast alongside if desired. This will make a great "Lunch Leftover" tomorrow.

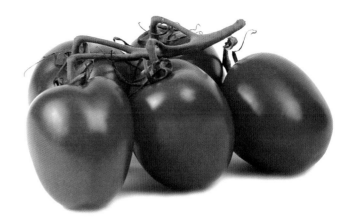

super-food salad with the perfect dressing

This has a refreshing zing and will keep well in the refrigerator (as long as it's not mixed with dressing). You may want to make this dressing again to use as a meat marinade or to toss on veggies before grilling.

Total time: 15 minutes

½ 12-ounce bag of rainbow slaw (also called California slaw or broccoli slaw), chopped slightly

1 pint cherry or grape tomatoes, halved

6 cups packed fresh baby spinach (5 ounces)

1 large garlic clove, peeled (alternatively, use garlic paste from a tube)

Fresh cracked pepper to taste

⅛ teaspoon salt

2 tablespoons lemon juice

1 tablespoon extra-virgin olive oil

1–2 fresh basil leaves, finely chopped (optional)

GROCERY LIST:
Rainbow slaw, also called California slaw or broccoli slaw (12-ounce bag)

Cherry or grape tomatoes (1 pint)

Fresh baby spinach (5 ounces)

Garlic clove (1)

Basil leaves (optional)

Salt

Fresh cracked black pepper

Lemon juice

Extra-virgin olive oil

1. In a large bowl, toss the first 3 salad ingredients.

2. Smash the garlic into a paste using a mortar and pestle, or simply mince the garlic and press it with the back of a spoon against the cutting board to form a paste. It may take a couple presses and a little muscle with the spoon to form the garlic paste, but it is worth the effort. (Smashing it into a paste helps the garlic distribute evenly within dressings and marinades).

3. Add salt and pepper to garlic paste and further process until well combined.

4. Mix the paste into a prep cup with lemon juice and olive oil. Add fresh basil, if desired, and mix well.

5. Drizzle the dressing over the vegetables and toss to coat. A small amount of this dressing has a lot of flavor, so use sparingly! If you have any extra dressing, it will keep in the refrigerator for up to a week.

Yield: 4 servings
(serving size: about 1¾ cups)

Nutrient Breakdown:
Calories 82

Fat 4g (1g saturated fat)

Cholesterol 0mg

Sodium 147mg

Carbohydrate 10g

Fiber 4g

Protein 4g

Plate Plan choices:
2 vegetables, 1 fat

pita chips

These are crunchy, tasty, and are a whole grain: a win-win-win! Use them to scoop up hummus dip or sprinkle them with cinnamon instead of savory seasonings when baking.

2 pita rounds (whole-wheat or oat bran)

2 teaspoons extra-virgin olive oil or Canola oil cooking spray

$1/8$ teaspoon Greek seasoning (such as Cavender's)

¼ teaspoon salt-free garlic and herb seasoning (such as Mrs. Dash)

GROCERY LIST:
2 pita rounds (whole-wheat or oat bran)

Greek Seasoning (such as Cavender's)

Salt-free garlic and herb seasoning (such as Mrs. Dash)

Extra-virgin olive oil

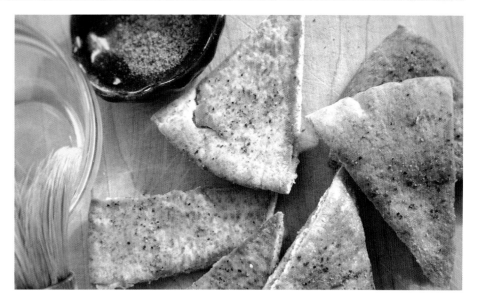

1. Preheat the oven to 400°F.
2. Brush each pita lightly with olive oil and sprinkle with seasonings (or spray lightly with canola oil cooking spray before sprinkling with seasonings).
3. Lay the pitas flat on a baking sheet and use a pizza cutter or clean kitchen shears to cut them into wedges.
4. Bake for 3–6 minutes. If the chips are not crispy all over, turn them and bake for 1–2 additional minutes.

Yield: 4 servings
(serving size: half a pita)

Nutrient Breakdown:
Calories 120

Fat 7g

Sodium 120mg

Carbohydrate 12g

Fiber 2g

Protein 2g

Plate Plan choices:
1 starch, 1 fat

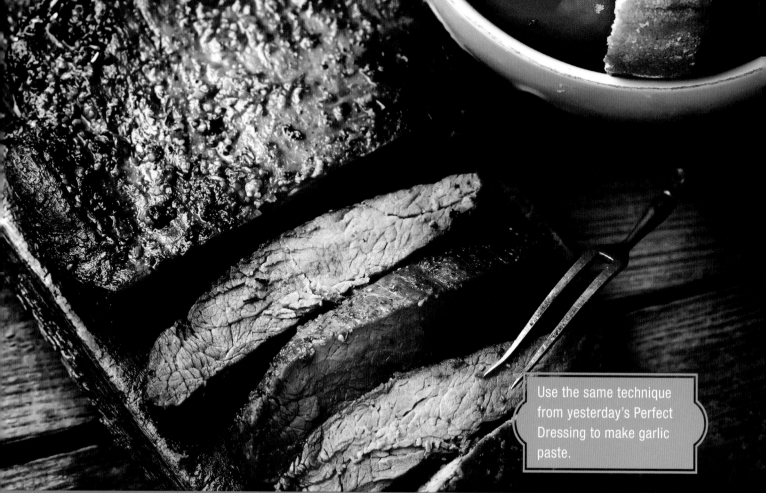

Use the same technique from yesterday's Perfect Dressing to make garlic paste.

DAY 27

Pricey Meal

grilled steak with garlic and lime

Lunch Leftovers

Today's meal has 3 recipes that serve 6 people and leaves you with leftover pasta salad to have later in the weekend. What great timing to invite guests over and show off some of your new recipes now that you are at about the halfway point of your Best Body Countdown journey!

Hands-on time: 25 minutes
Total time: 55 minutes (includes 30 minutes marinating time)

1½ pounds flat iron or flank steak

¼ cup lime juice (from 2 limes)

4 cloves garlic, smashed into a paste (or use garlic paste from a tube)

1 tablespoon reduced-sodium soy sauce

2 teaspoons extra-virgin olive oil

Canola oil cooking spray

Cracked black pepper, if desired

GROCERY LIST:
Lime juice (¼ cup)

Garlic cloves (4)

Flat iron or flank steak (1½ pounds)

Reduced-sodium soy sauce

Extra-virgin olive oil

Canola oil cooking spray

Cracked black pepper

Salt-free garlic and herb seasoning (such as Mrs. Dash)

Extra-virgin olive oil

1. Remove all visible fat and silver skin from meat. To remove the silver skin (a tough membrane with an iridescent hue), slip a knife blade between the silver skin and meat, angle the knife slightly upward, and use a gentle back-and-forth sawing motion to cut away the membrane.

2. In a large plastic zip-top bag or glass baking dish, combine the lime juice, garlic, soy sauce, and oil. Swish the bag or whisk to combine. Add the meat and turn to coat. Seal the bag or cover the dish and refrigerate for 30 minutes or up to several hours, turning meat occasionally.

3. If using an outdoor grill, preheat grill on medium-high. If using a ridged stovetop grill pan, lightly spray with cooking spray.

4. Remove meat from bag and sprinkle with pepper, if desired. Discard the marinade. Cook the meat over medium-high heat for 6–7 minutes on each side until an internal temperature of 145°F on a meat thermometer is reached, or until the desired doneness is achieved (to maintain its tenderness, do not overcook this cut of meat).

5. Transfer to a cutting board. Let stand for 5 minutes. Cut diagonally across the grain into very thin slices.

Yield: 6 servings
(serving size: 3 ounces)

Nutrient Breakdown:
Calories 230

Fat 10g (4g saturated fat)

Cholesterol 60mg

Sodium 190mg

Carbohydrate 2g

Fiber 0g

Protein 32g

Plate Plan choices:
3 lean meats

Leftover steak is great over the Mexican Slaw from Day 25. Yum! Also, consider grilled pineapple as a dessert with a lime-honey drizzle, or yogurt with lime and honey.

roasted or grilled cabbage

Total time: 15 minutes

Club Favorite

If you have never loved cabbage, this is the recipe for you! Roasting the cabbage gives it a deliciously sweet, nutty flavor. Grilling it takes it one step further and adds a smoky char flavor. It is a great change to grill your vegetables, especially if you already have the grill going.

This recipe uses a whole head of cabbage, but if you won't use 8 servings, feel free to reduce the recipe by half and chop the extra cabbage to mix into the green salad suggested as a side for tomorrow's meal.

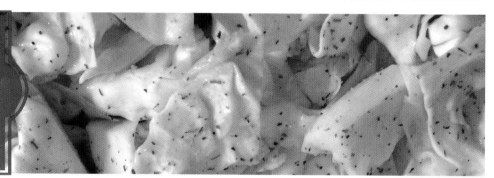

Canola oil cooking spray

1 head of green cabbage

2 tablespoons extra-virgin olive oil

1 teaspoon Jane's Krazy Mixed-Up Salt

¼ teaspoon black pepper

½ teaspoon dried thyme (optional)

Lemon wedges or a drizzle of juice (optional)

GROCERY LIST:
Head of green cabbage (1)

Lemon juice (optional)

Jane's Krazy Mixed-Up Salt

Black pepper

Dried thyme (optional)

Extra-virgin olive oil

Canola oil cooking spray

1. Preheat the oven to 425°F. Line a large baking sheet with aluminum foil and spray with cooking spray.

2. Cut the cabbage in half (from the top down through the stem end) and then cut each half into quarters (making 8 wedges). Carefully cut the tough center core out of each wedge and place the cabbage wedges on the baking sheet in a single layer.

3. Combine the olive oil, salt, pepper and thyme (if using) in a small bowl. Using a pastry brush, lightly brush each wedge with the oil mixture.

4. Roast for 15 minutes, then flip the wedges over (using tongs may help keep the wedges together, however they may fall apart at this point, which is to be expected). Roast for another 12 to 15 minutes until slightly brown and tender. Serve with lemon, if desired.

Yield: 8 servings
(serving size: 1 wedge or ½ cup chopped cabbage)

Nutrient Breakdown:
Calories 60

Fat 3.5g (0.5g saturated fat)

Cholesterol 0mg

Sodium 150mg

Carbohydrate 6g

Fiber 3g

Protein 1g

Plate Plan choices:
1½ vegetables, 1 fat

TO GRILL: Prepare cabbage as above through step 3, and then put the cabbage in a vegetable-grilling pan (do not over-crowd). Expect the cabbage to fall apart a little. Grill the cabbage over medium-low heat for 10 minutes (or until done). Stir to rotate cabbage about half way through the cooking process. Serve with lemon, if desired.

edamame pasta salad

Hands-on time: 25 minutes
Total time: 1 hour 25 minutes
(includes refrigerator time)

Quicker-Fix   Lunch Leftovers

This pasta salad has a rainbow of colors and will be a welcome addition to weekday lunches or festive gatherings anytime of the year. This makes a lot of food to enjoy with others on the weekend!

2 cups whole-wheat penne pasta (6 ounces)

1 16-ounce package shelled edamame (typically found in the freezer case)

⅔ cup chopped red onion

1 medium zucchini, chopped

½ medium red bell pepper, chopped

1 pint cherry tomatoes, halved or quartered

Dressing
3 tablespoons balsamic vinegar

2 tablespoons extra-virgin olive oil

2 teaspoons lemon juice

¾ teaspoon dried dill weed

½ teaspoon dried oregano leaves

1 teaspoon Greek seasoning (such as Cavender's)

Fresh cracked black pepper, to taste

1 cup crumbled feta cheese (4 ounces)

Parsley (optional)

1. Cook the pasta according to package directions (omitting the salt and oil). During the last 5 minutes of cooking, add the edamame to the pasta pot and bring back to a boil for 5 minutes. Drain pasta mixture and rinse with cool water.

2. Combine pasta in a large bowl with remaining vegetables (red onion through tomatoes).

3. In a separate bowl, whisk together the dressing ingredients (balsamic vinegar through black pepper). Pour dressing over pasta mixture and toss to coat. Add feta cheese and toss again.

4. Chill for 1–2 hours before serving. Toss before serving to re-coat the salad with dressing, as it will sink to the bottom a bit. Sprinkle with parsley garnish if desired.

Yield: 10 servings
(serving size: 1 cup)

Nutrient Breakdown:
Calories 180

Fat 8g (2g saturated fat)

Cholesterol 0mg

Sodium 270mg

Carbohydrate 19g

Fiber 5g

Protein 9g

Plate Plan choices: 1 starch, 1 vegetable, 1 lean meat

GROCERY LIST:
Red onion (⅔ cup chopped)

Zucchini (1 medium)

Red bell pepper (1)

Cherry tomatoes (1 pint)

Lemon juice

Parsley (optional)

Whole-wheat penne pasta (6 ounces or 2 cups)

Shelled edamame (16 ounces or 3 cups, typically found in the freezer case)

Crumbled feta cheese (1 cup)

Balsamic vinegar

Extra-virgin olive oil

Dried dill weed

Dried oregano leaves

Greek seasoning (such as Cavender's)

Cracked black pepper

 COUNTDOWN QUICKER-FIX:

Use 6 tablespoons of Newman's Own Balsamic Vinaigrette dressing plus dill instead of making your own dressing (the nutrient content for this one is very similar). The Countdown Quicker-Fix method works in a pinch, but the flavor of this homemade dressing is superior, lower in sugar, and really only takes about 5 minutes to make. Either way, this salad makes a great side dish or "Lunch Leftover:" try serving it over a bed of lettuce with grilled chicken on top. Delish!

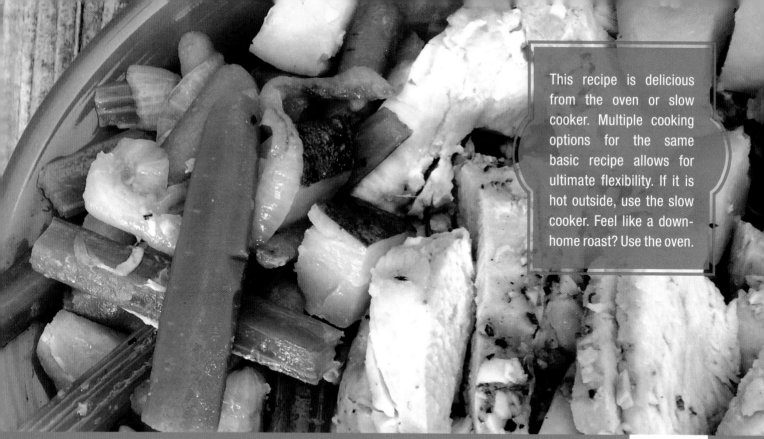

This recipe is delicious from the oven or slow cooker. Multiple cooking options for the same basic recipe allows for ultimate flexibility. If it is hot outside, use the slow cooker. Feel like a down-home roast? Use the oven.

DAY 26

Slow-Cooker
Optional

one-dish roasted turkey dinner

Lunch Leftovers

Cooking a large serving of lean meat on the weekend helps to create grab-and-go or quick meals throughout the week. Tomorrow's Turkey Enchilada Casserole recipe turns leftover turkey into a wholesome planned-over. Slices of turkey breast also make a great addition to a main-dish salad anytime.

suggested side: green salad

Hands-on time: 20 minutes
Total time: 1 hour 20 minutes
(if using the oven)

 *The turkey breast takes 2 days in the refrigerator to thaw.

To make in the slow cooker: Spray the crock of a slow cooker with cooking spray, add vegetables, half the oil, garlic-salt mixture, and toss to coat. Prepare the turkey as above and place on top of the vegetables. Cover with the slow-cooker lid and cook on low for 8–10 hours.

Canola oil cooking spray

2 tablespoons extra-virgin olive oil, divided

1 tablespoon Jane's Krazy Mixed-Up Salt, divided

4 garlic cloves, minced and divided

1 pound potatoes (any variety), cut into large bite-sized pieces with skin

½ pound baby carrots or peeled whole carrots, cut into 1-inch pieces, thick pieces halved

2 medium onions, sliced

4 stalks of celery, cut into 1-inch pieces

3 pounds frozen boneless turkey breast* (frozen turkey: thawed and gravy pack removed)

Chopped parsley (optional garnish)

1. Preheat the oven to 350°F. Cover a large roasting pan (or a 9x13-inch pan) with aluminum foil and coat with cooking spray. Place 1 tablespoon of oil, 1 teaspoon seasoning salt, and half of the garlic on the prepared pan, add the vegetables (potatoes through celery), and toss to coat evenly with oil and seasoning.

2. Combine the remaining salt, oil, and garlic in a small bowl. Rub this mixture under the skin of the turkey, pressing it into the meat.

3. Place the turkey on top of the vegetables and seal with foil. Place in the oven and cook for 1 hour or until done (turkey is done when an internal temperature of 165°F is reached on a meat thermometer).

Yield: 6 servings
(serving size: 3 ounces of turkey and ¾ cup vegetables, plus save about 1 pound turkey for recipes)

Nutrient Breakdown:
Calories 250

Fat 6g
(0.5g saturated fat,
2g monounsaturated fat)

Cholesterol 45mg

Sodium 620mg

Carbohydrate 21g

Fiber 3g

Protein 30g

Plate Plan choices:
1 starch, 2 vegetables,
4 very lean meats

GROCERY LIST:
Garlic cloves (4)

Potatoes (1 pound, any variety)

Baby carrots or whole carrots (½ pound)

Onions (2 medium)

Celery (4 stalks)

Parsley (optional garnish)

Boneless turkey breast (3 pounds frozen turkey)

Jane's Krazy Mixed-Up Salt

Extra-virgin olive oil

Canola oil cooking spray

Salad fixings (suggested side)

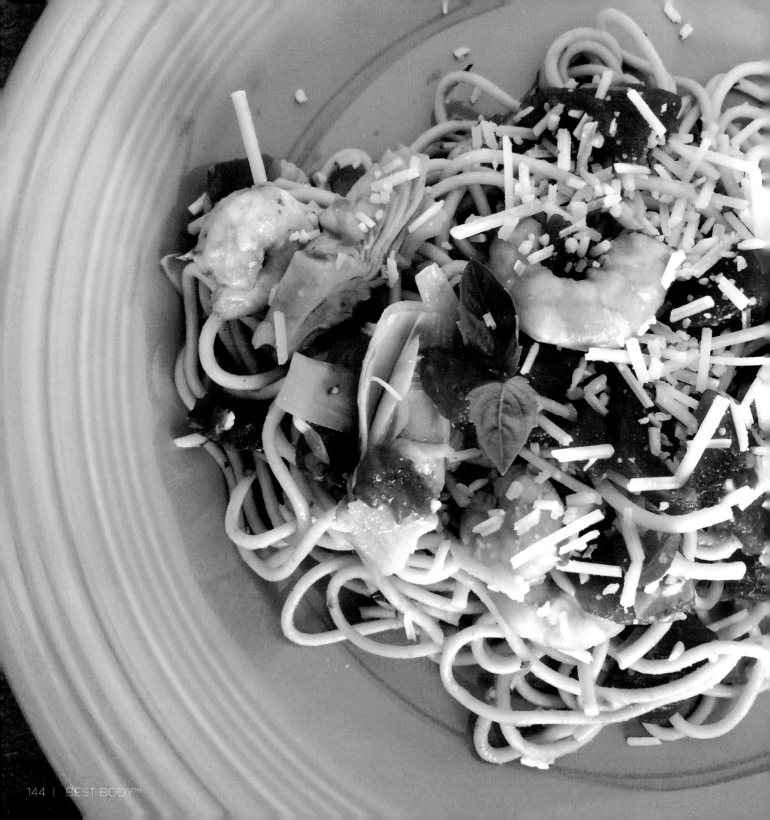

recipes & menu:
week five

> "Strength is the capacity to break a chocolate bar into four pieces with your bare hands and then eat just one of the pieces."
>
> —JUDITH VIORST

menu key:

Lunch Leftovers

Pricey Meal

Quicker-Fix

Slow-Cooker

Club Favorite

Easy Meal

DAY 25
Turkey Enchilada Casserole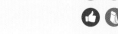
Mexican Slaw

DAY 24
Vegetarian Chili
Roasted Cauliflower with Paprika
Suggested side: raw veggies and dip

DAY 23
Pasta with Artichokes and Shrimp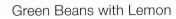
Sweet and Simple Spinach Salad

DAY 22
Southwestern Chopped Salad

DAY 21
Sesame-Crusted Tuna Steak
Green Beans with Lemon
Suggested side: brown rice

DAY 20
Broiled Chicken with Herbs
Pasta Salad Florentine
Suggested side: broccoli

DAY 19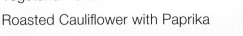
Easy Slow-Cooker Beef Roast Dinner
Suggested side: green salad
Whole grain rolls (if needed)

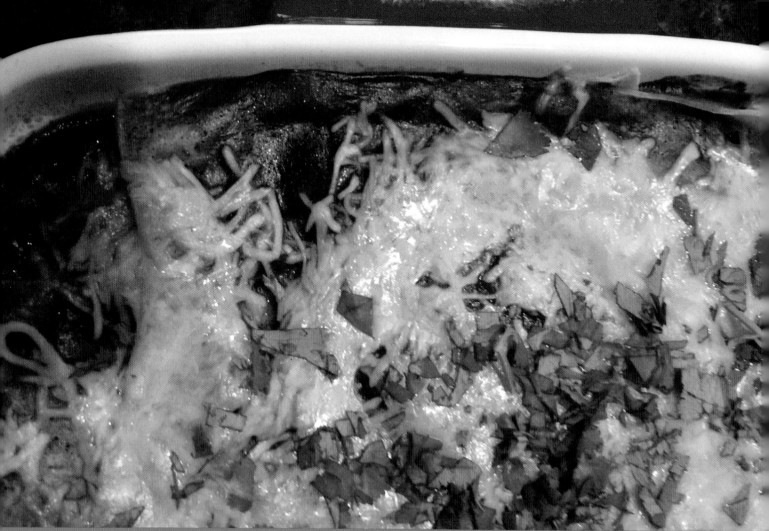

DAY 25

turkey enchilada casserole

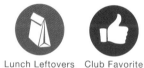

Lunch Leftovers   Club Favorite

This is a great use of leftover turkey (or chicken) and an easy way to get your Mexican food fix at home, where the bottomless baskets of chips aren't there to tempt you.

Hands-on time: 20 minutes   Total time: 50 total minutes

Canola oil cooking spray

2 teaspoons extra-virgin olive oil

1 small onion, chopped (about 1 cup)

½ green bell pepper, chopped (about ½ cup)

2 cloves garlic, minced

2 cups chopped roasted turkey (or chicken) breast

½ cup salsa

1 14.5-ounce can of pinto beans, drained and rinsed

2 teaspoons chili powder

½ cup plain, nonfat Greek yogurt

1 cup (4 ounces) shredded reduced-fat Mexican cheese, divided

11 6-inch corn tortillas

1 10-ounce can enchilada sauce

Fresh cilantro (optional, but delicious garnish)

Lime (optional)

1. Preheat the oven to 350°F. Spray a large nonstick skillet with cooking spray, add oil, and place over medium heat. Once the oil is hot, add onion, green pepper, and garlic. Sauté until tender (about 3 minutes).

2. Add turkey, salsa, beans, and chili powder. Stir to combine and cook for 3 minutes. Remove pan from heat. Add yogurt and ½ cup of cheese, mix, and set aside.

3. Prepare tortillas by cutting 10 tortillas in half (the 11th will remain whole). Line the bottom of a 9x9-inch baking pan by placing 7 halves (cut sides facing out) around the bottom of the pan and one of the halves covering the space in the middle. Then layer following these directions:
   · Layer half of the turkey mixture on top of the tortillas
   · Pour one-third of the enchilada sauce over the turkey
   · Repeat the tortilla layer using 7 tortilla halves
   · Add remaining turkey mixture
   · Pour one-third of the enchilada sauce over the turkey mixture
   · Cover the last layer with tortillas, leaving the middle tortilla whole
   · Top with the remaining sauce
   · Cover with aluminum foil and bake for 30 minutes.

4. Uncover the casserole, top with the remaining ½ cup cheese, and bake an additional 5 minutes. Allow casserole to set for 15 minutes before cutting into 6 equal pieces. Serve with cilantro and lime if desired.

Yield: 6 servings
(serving size: 1 piece)

Nutrient Breakdown:
Calories 390

Fat 10g (3g saturated fat)

Cholesterol 50mg

Sodium 650mg

Carbohydrate 45g

Fiber 6g

Protein 28g

Plate Plan choices:
2 starches,
2 vegetables,
3 lean meats

GROCERY LIST:
Onion (1 small, chopped)

Green bell pepper (½ cup chopped)

Garlic cloves (2)

Fresh cilantro (optional)

Lime (optional wedges for serving)

Turkey or chicken (2 cups, precooked)

6-inch corn tortillas (11)

Pinto beans (1 14.5-ounce can)

Enchilada sauce (1 10-ounce can)

Salsa

Plain, nonfat Greek yogurt

Shredded reduced-fat Mexican cheese

Chili powder

Extra-virgin olive oil

Canola oil cooking spray

For even bigger flavor, add ¼ teaspoon chipotle chili powder when you add the regular chili powder.

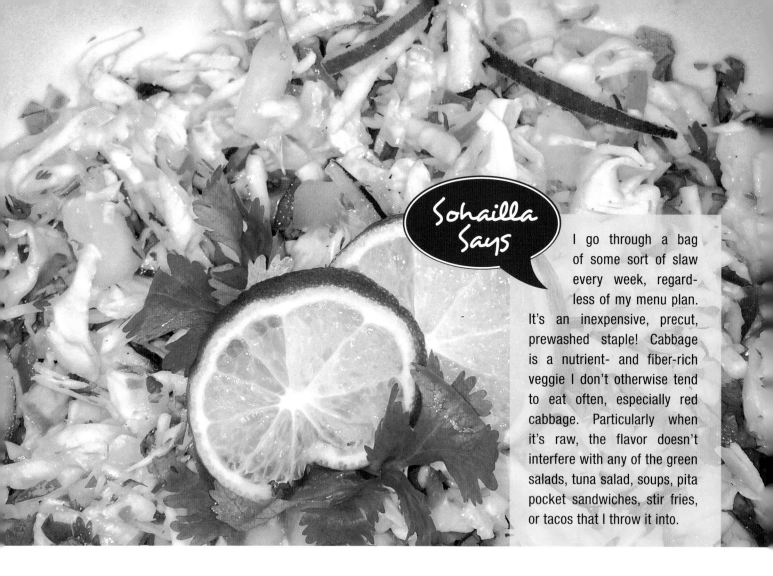

mexican slaw

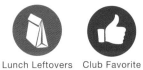

Lunch Leftovers   Club Favorite

This is both fresh and zesty! It pairs well with Mexican cuisine and is also great with grilled steak or chicken.

Hands-on time: 15 minutes
Total time: 2 hours and 15 minutes (includes refrigerator time)

2–3 tablespoons fresh lime juice, divided

1 tablespoon extra-virgin olive oil

¼ teaspoon of salt

¼ teaspoon black pepper

1 cup chopped frozen or fresh mango

1 16-ounce bag of slaw mix

½ cup coarsely chopped fresh cilantro (not optional in this recipe)

1 tablespoon chopped jalapeno (fresh or jarred)

¼ cup finely sliced red onion

GROCERY LIST:

Slaw mix (16-ounce bag)

Jalapeño, fresh or jarred

Red onion

Lime juice (2–3 tablespoons)

Fresh cilantro

Frozen or fresh mango

Salt

Black pepper

Extra-virgin olive oil

1. Combine 2 tablespoons lime juice, olive oil, salt, pepper, and mango in a bowl. Set aside.
2. In a large bowl, combine slaw mix, cilantro, jalapeño, and onion.
3. Pour dressing over slaw mix and refrigerate for 1–2 hours so flavors combine. Add more lime juice if needed. Serve chilled.

Yield: 6 servings
(serving size: 1 cup)

Nutrient Breakdown:
Calories 80

Fat 2.5g (0g saturated fat)

Cholesterol 0mg

Sodium 125mg

Carbohydrate 14g

Fiber 4g

Protein 2g

Plate Plan choices:
2 vegetables

Kim's Comment

Slaws are best when made the night before and left to sit in the refrigerator, though you can just make this while the Turkey Enchilada Casserole is baking. If you have extra mango, use it to make tropical smoothies or as a topping for yogurt. (Greek yogurt + vanilla extract + mango + almonds = Yum!)

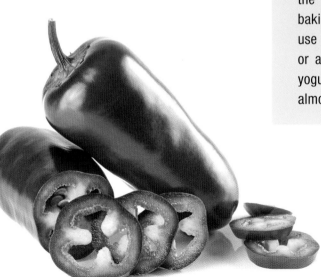

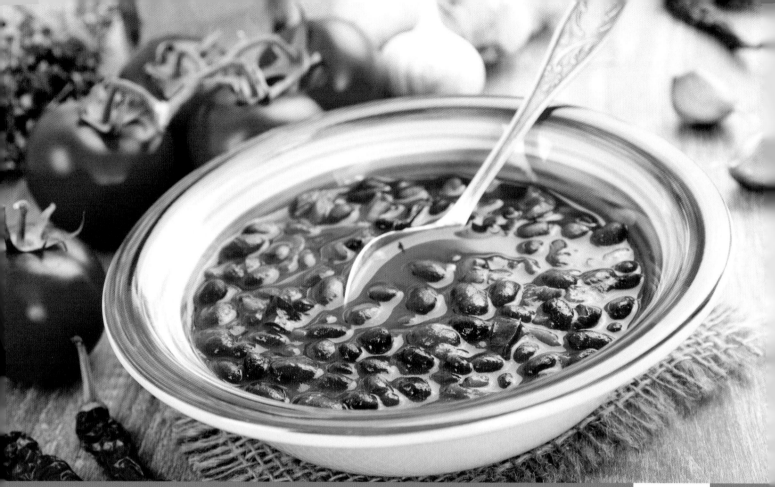

DAY 24

Slow-Cooker

vegetarian chili

Lunch Leftovers

You will not notice the absence of meat here. This chili is mild, so feel free to spice it up by adding any of the following: crushed red pepper flakes, cayenne pepper, or chopped chipotle peppers. The recipe makes a lot, so plan on "Lunch Leftovers!"

suggested side: raw veggies and
yogurt-based dressing for dipping

Hands-on time: 20 minutes
Total time: 8 hours and 15 minutes

Tofu is packed in water, and many recipes will tell you to drain and press the water out of tofu. This is actually an important step because removing the water allows the tofu to absorb the flavors of the recipe. In this chili recipe, instead of pressing the water out, the water is cooked out, which is more effective when using crumbled tofu.

1 tablespoon extra-virgin olive oil

1 12-ounce bag frozen Cajun-style mirepoix blend (onion, green pepper, celery)

4 garlic cloves, minced

1 14-ounce package firm organic tofu, drained

1 cup unsalted vegetable broth

1 medium zucchini, finely chopped

1 14.5-ounce can crushed tomatoes

1 14.5-ounce can fire-roasted diced tomatoes

1 15-ounce can reduced-sodium black beans, drained and rinsed (or precooked beans)

1 15-ounce can reduced-sodium kidney beans, drained and rinsed

2 tablespoons chili powder

1 teaspoon ground cumin

1 teaspoon dried oregano

¼ teaspoon salt

1 cup plain, nonfat Greek yogurt

1 cup reduced-fat shredded cheddar cheese

1. Add oil to a large nonstick skillet and place over medium-high heat. Once hot, add the frozen vegetables, garlic, and tofu (you'll want to break up the tofu by squishing it between your fingers into the pan: it's easy and effective). Cook the veggies and tofu until most of the water has evaporated from the pan (8–10 minutes).

2. Meanwhile, add the broth, zucchini, tomatoes, beans and remaining spices to the slow cooker. Add the prepared tofu mixture to the slow cooker, stirring to combine. Cover and cook on low for 8–10 hours.

3. Serve with 2 tablespoons each of Greek yogurt and cheese.

Yield: 8 servings
(serving size: 1¼ cup chili and 2 tablespoons each of Greek yogurt and cheese)

Nutrient Breakdown:
Calories 250

Fat 6g (2g saturated fat, 1g monounsaturated fat)

Cholesterol 10mg

Sodium 570mg

Carbohydrate 31g

Fiber 9g

Protein 19g

Plate Plan choices:
1½ starches, 2 vegetables, 2 lean meats/protein

GROCERY LIST:
Zucchini (1 medium)

Garlic cloves (4)

Firm organic tofu (14-ounce package)

Unsalted vegetable broth

Crushed tomatoes (14.5-ounce can)

Fire-roasted diced tomatoes (14.5-ounce can)

Reduced-sodium black beans (15-ounce can)

Reduced-sodium kidney beans (15-ounce can)

Plain, nonfat Greek yogurt

Reduced-fat shredded cheddar cheese

Frozen Cajun-style mirepoix blend (12-ounce bag)

Chili powder

Ground cumin

Dried oregano

Salt

Extra-virgin olive oil

Raw veggies (suggested side)

Greek yogurt-based ranch dressing such as Bolthouse Farms (dip for suggested side)

roasted cauliflower with paprika

Hands-on time: 12 minutes
Total time: 22 minutes

Lunch Leftovers

Cauliflower is traditionally under-utilized, but the rich taste you'll get from roasting this vegetable will have you adding it to your regular menu rotation. Roasting brings out the natural sweetness and boosts the flavor. This makes 8 servings, so if you don't plan to use that much, you may want to get a 12-ounce bag of precut florets and reduce the other ingredients listed by half.

Canola oil cooking spray

2 tablespoons extra-virgin olive oil

1 teaspoon Jane's Krazy Mixed-Up Salt

¼ teaspoon black pepper

½ teaspoon paprika (or alternate seasoning options)

1 head cauliflower, cut into bite-sized florets

1 tablespoon chopped fresh parsley (optional)

Lemon wedges (optional, but delicious)

GROCERY LIST:
Cauliflower (1 medium head or one 12-ounce bag of florets if halving recipe)

Fresh parsley (optional)

Lemon (optional wedges for serving)

Jane's Krazy Mixed-Up Salt

Black pepper

Paprika (or alternate seasoning option)

Extra-virgin olive oil

Canola oil cooking spray

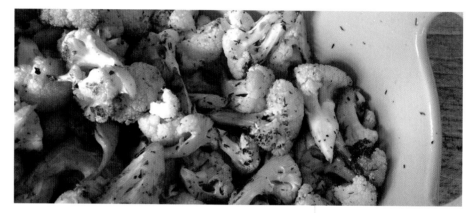

1. Preheat the oven to 425°F. Line a large baking pan with aluminum foil (for easy clean up) and spray with cooking spray.

2. Pour the oil, salt, pepper, and paprika onto the prepared pan. Add cauliflower and toss to evenly coat with oil. Once mixed, spread the cauliflower out in a single layer on the baking sheet.

3. Roast for 20–24 minutes, stirring or turning halfway through the cooking time to promote even browning.

Yield: 8 servings
(serving size: ½ cup)

Nutrient Breakdown:
Calories 50

Fat 3.5g (0.5g saturated fat)

Cholesterol 0mg

Sodium 160mg

Carbohydrate 4g

Fiber 2g

Protein 2g

Plate Plan choices:
1 vegetable, 1 fat

ALTERNATE SEASONINGS:
½ teaspoon dried thyme + parsley + lemon

½ teaspoon dried dill + parsley + lemon

½ teaspoon cumin + cilantro + lime juice

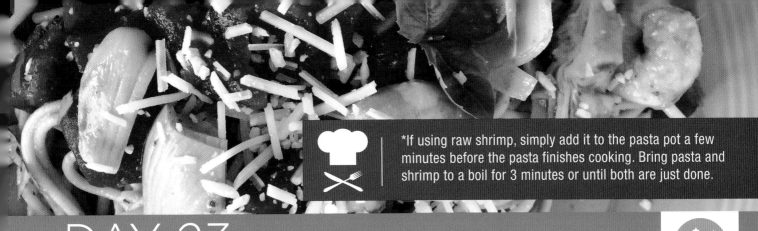

*If using raw shrimp, simply add it to the pasta pot a few minutes before the pasta finishes cooking. Bring pasta and shrimp to a boil for 3 minutes or until both are just done.

DAY 23

pasta with artichokes and shrimp

Easy Meal

Total time: 25 minutes

Club Favorite

This meal uses pantry staples and can be thrown together quickly. Add a side salad and you will be well on your way to meeting your vegetable quota for the day.

suggested side: spinach salad

6 ounces whole-wheat spaghetti

1 6-ounce jar marinated artichoke hearts, undrained

1 14.5-ounce can no-salt-added diced tomatoes

1 pound cooked or raw* shrimp

½ teaspoon Italian seasoning

2 tablespoons shredded Parmesan cheese

Fresh basil leaves (optional garnish)

GROCERY LIST:
Fresh basil (optional garnish)

Shrimp (1 pound cooked, or raw*)

Whole-wheat spaghetti (6 ounces)

Marinated artichoke hearts (6-ounce jar)

No-salt-added diced tomatoes (14.5-ounce can)

Shredded Parmesan cheese

Italian seasoning

1. Cook the pasta according to the package directions (omitting salt).

2. Meanwhile, pour the artichoke hearts into a medium saucepan and cut them into smaller pieces using clean kitchen shears (cutting them in the pan minimizes clean up). Add the can of tomatoes to the pan, chopping the tomatoes with the kitchen shears a little as well.

3. Stir in the shrimp and Italian seasoning, bring to a boil, and then reduce heat to low. Simmer until heated thoroughly.

4. Once pasta is done, drain and serve with the prepared sauce. Top with Parmesan cheese and garnish with basil if desired.

Yield: 4 servings
(serving size: ¾ cup pasta, 3 ounces shrimp, and ½ cup of the sauce)

Nutrient Breakdown:
Calories 268

Fat 4g
(1.5g saturated fat)

Cholesterol 150mg

Sodium 430mg

Carbohydrate 41g

Fiber 6g

Protein 21g

Plate Plan choices:
2 starches,
2 vegetables,
3 very lean meats

sweet and simple spinach salad

Total time: 10 minutes

When you only have a few minutes and need to round out a meal, this is a sweet and simple way to do it!

¼ cup walnuts, coarsely chopped and toasted

6 cups packed fresh baby spinach (5 ounces)

1½ cups of strawberries, sliced

3½ tablespoons balsamic vinaigrette (such as Newman's Own)

GROCERY LIST:
Walnuts (¼ cup)

Fresh baby spinach (5 ounces)

Strawberries (1½ cups)

Balsamic vinaigrette (such as Newman's Own)

1. To toast nuts: place a dry, nonstick skillet over medium heat and add nuts. Toast the nuts for 2–4 minutes, stirring or shaking the pan frequently to avoid burning. As they become fragrant and begin to change color, remove them from the heat.

2. In a large bowl, gently toss the spinach and strawberries with vinaigrette and add the nuts to serve.

Yield: 4 servings
(serving size: about 1¾ cups)

Nutrient Breakdown:
Calories 110

Fat 8g (1g saturated fat)

Sodium 260mg

Carbohydrate 11g

Fiber 3g

Protein 2g

Plate Plan choices:
1 vegetable, ½ fruit, 1 fat

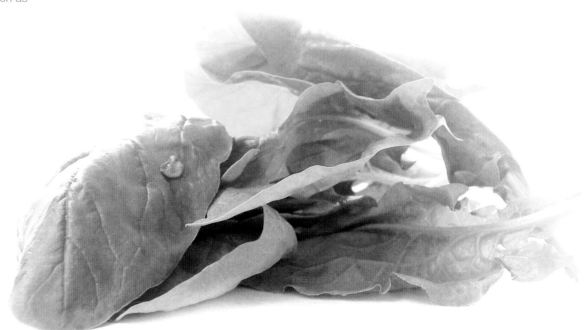

Easy Meal

southwestern chopped salad

Instead of steak and potato, how about steak and salad…it is tastier than you'd think! Try it! This is a fairly low-calorie meal, so you could consider adding a serving of tortilla chips, but only if you know you won't overdo it on that bag later. A piece of fruit is a good add-on option, too.

Hands-on time: 20 minutes
Total time: 2 hours and 15 minutes (includes 2 hours marinating time)

1 pound sirloin steak

2 tablespoons salt-free chipotle seasoning (such as Mrs. Dash)

½ tablespoon extra-virgin olive oil

1 10-ounce bag Southwest chopped salad mix (such as Taylor Farms or Dole)

½ cup reduced-fat cheddar cheese, shredded

1 can reduced-sodium black beans, rinsed and drained (or 1½ cups precooked beans)

GROCERY LIST:
Southwest chopped salad mix (10-ounce bag, such as Taylor Farms or Dole)

Sirloin steak (1 pound)

Reduced-sodium black beans (15-ounce can)

Reduced-fat shredded cheddar cheese

Salt-free chipotle seasoning (such as Mrs. Dash)

Extra virgin olive oil

Tortilla chips (cautiously suggested side)

1. Cut steak into thin strips and place in a gallon-size plastic zip-top bag with seasoning and oil. Let most of the air out of the bag while zipping it. Knead the steak and seasoning gently so that the marinade covers the meat. Allow steak to marinate for 2 hours in the refrigerator or overnight if possible.

2. Remove the dressing packet from the salad and set aside. Combine the chopped salad, cheese, and beans in a large bowl.

3. Toss the salad with half to two-thirds of the dressing from the packet. (It is best not to use the entire packet of dressing from the salad bag because it's typically high in fat and calories.) Alternatively, you can use a separate reduced fat Southwest-style dressing if desired.

4. Place a nonstick skillet over medium heat. Once hot, add beef and marinade to the pan (the pan should not need oil because of the marinade). Sauté the beef for 3–5 minutes, leaving a little pink in the center. Serve warm or cold over the salad.

Yield: 4 servings
(serving size: about 1¾ cups)

Nutrient Breakdown:
(includes two-thirds of the dressing packet):
Calories 330

Fat 16g
(6g saturated fat)

Sodium 440mg

Carbohydrate 21g

Fiber 7g

Protein 33g

Plate Plan choices:
1 starch,
2 vegetables,
4 lean meats, 1 fat

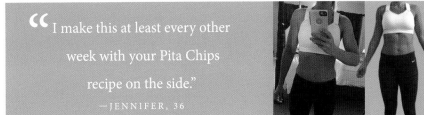

" I make this at least every other week with your Pita Chips recipe on the side."
—JENNIFER, 36

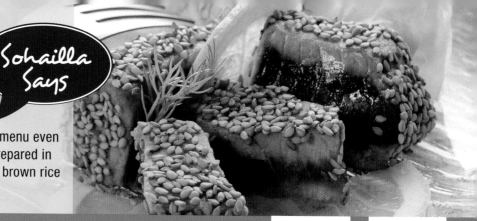

This is my very favorite dish to order when out to eat, especially when visiting the coast. If you've never tried tuna steak, trust me, it is nothing like tuna from a can. I love today's menu even more considering the whole meal can be prepared in less than 20 minutes (if you use precooked brown rice or the quick-cook variety).

Sohailla Says

DAY 21

Easy Meal

Pricey Meal

sesame-crusted tuna steak

This is definitely a special-occasion meal, but we think you deserve it... enjoy!

suggested side: brown rice

Total time: 12 minutes

1 12-ounce package chopped Asian-blend salad (such as Dole)

4 sashimi-grade tuna steaks (about 1¼–1½ pounds)

⅓ cup sesame seeds

Canola oil cooking spray

1 tablespoon canola oil

GROCERY LIST:

Chopped Asian-blend salad such as Dole or similar (12-ounce package)

4 sashimi-grade tuna steaks (1¼-1½ pounds)

Sesame seeds (⅓ cup, using both plain and black seeds looks nice)

Canola oil

1. Place 2 tablespoons of the dressing packet provided in the Asian blend into a bowl and brush over both sides of the tuna.

2. Pour the sesame seeds onto a dinner plate and dip the tuna steaks into the seeds to press some onto each side.

3. Coat a nonstick skillet with cooking spray and add oil, then place over medium-high heat. Once the oil is hot, swirl to coat the pan and add tuna, 2 steaks at a time. Sear for 90 seconds on one side and 60 seconds on the other side for a rare tuna steak (recommended). We suggest using a timer.

4. Toss the salad from the bag with the rest of the dressing provided; serve with the tuna steak on top.

Yield: 4 servings
(4 4½-ounce servings of tuna steak and 1 cup salad)

Nutrient Breakdown:
Calories 400

Fat 22g (3.5g saturated fat, 1100mg omega-3 fatty acids)

Cholesterol 55mg

Sodium 270mg

Carbohydrate 12g

Added sugar 5g from dressing

Fiber 3g

Protein 37g

Plate Plan choices:
5 lean meats, 1½ vegetables, 2 fats

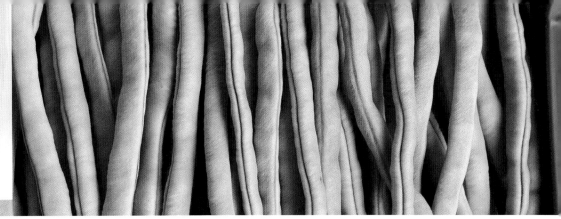

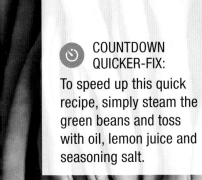

⏱ COUNTDOWN
QUICKER-FIX:

To speed up this quick recipe, simply steam the green beans and toss with oil, lemon juice and seasoning salt.

green beans with lemon

Hands-on time: 7 minutes

Quicker-Fix

The lemon juice brightens and flavors these green beans in a flash. A tried-and-true seasoning technique for almost any vegetable is olive oil, lemon juice, plus salt or other seasoning. Try this with a few sliced tomatoes thrown in for added color.

1 12-ounce microwavable package of green beans

½ tablespoon extra-virgin olive oil

2 garlic cloves, minced

½ teaspoon Jane's Krazy Mixed-Up Salt

1 tablespoon lemon juice

GROCERY LIST:
Fresh green beans
(12-ounce microwavable package)

Garlic cloves (2)

Lemon juice
(1 tablespoon)

Jane's Krazy Mixed-Up salt

Extra-virgin olive oil

1. Steam green beans (either as directed on package or in a microwave-safe bowl). To steam green beans in a bowl, place clean, trimmed green beans in a microwave-safe bowl, add ¼ cup water, and cover with a damp paper towel. Microwave for 2–4 minutes (depending on how tender you like your green beans).

2. Add oil to a large nonstick skillet and place over medium-high heat. Once the oil is hot, add the garlic and cook for 30 seconds, then add the drained green beans. Add the salt and stir to combine.

3. Transfer the beans to a serving dish and drizzle with lemon juice.

Yield: 4 servings
(serving size: 1 cup)

Nutrient Breakdown:
Calories 45

Fat 2g

Cholesterol 0mg

Sodium 150mg

Carbohydrate 7g

Fiber 2g

Protein 2g

Plate Plan choices:
2 vegetables

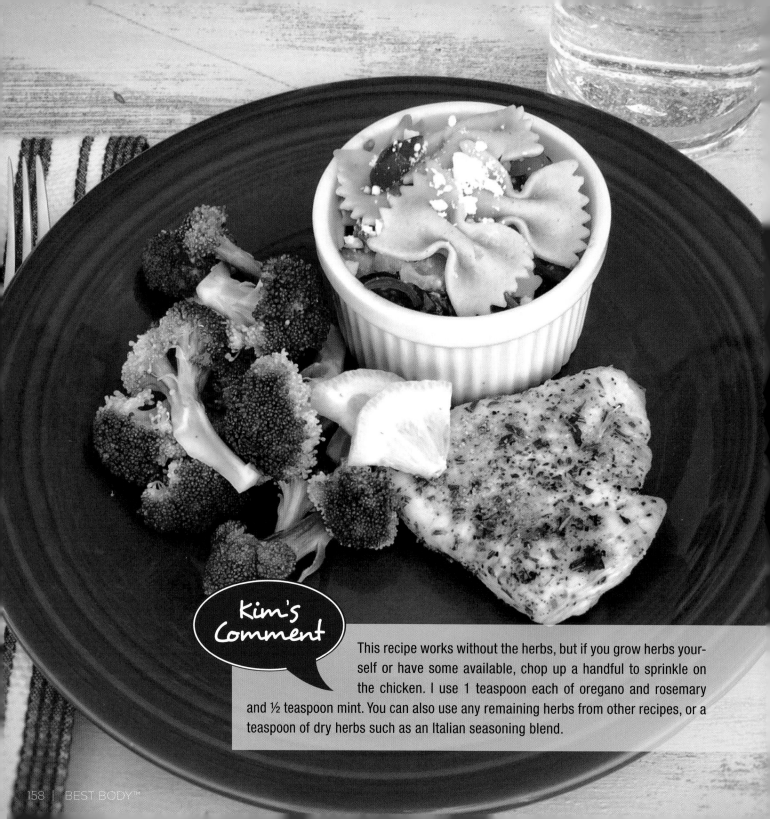

Kim's Comment

This recipe works without the herbs, but if you grow herbs yourself or have some available, chop up a handful to sprinkle on the chicken. I use 1 teaspoon each of oregano and rosemary and ½ teaspoon mint. You can also use any remaining herbs from other recipes, or a teaspoon of dry herbs such as an Italian seasoning blend.

DAY 20

broiled chicken with herbs

Lunch Leftovers

For a simple meal, try this basic broiled chicken recipe. Pair it with veggies the first night and use the leftovers on a sandwich, in a soup, or on top of salad. To be sure you have extra, simply double (or triple) the recipe and freeze! In fact, you may want to double this recipe and leave the herbs off of a couple chicken breasts so that you can freeze* them to use on Day 15's Chicken and Bok Choy Stir-fry.

suggested side: steamed or sautéed broccoli

Hands-on time: 10 minutes
Total time: 20 minutes

1½ pounds boneless, skinless chicken breasts

1 tablespoon extra-virgin olive oil

1 tablespoon grilled chicken seasoning blend

2½ teaspoons chopped fresh herbs of choice or 1 teaspoon dried herbs of choice

GROCERY LIST:
Boneless, skinless chicken breasts (1½ pounds)

Grilled chicken seasoning

Herbs of choice (if desired)

Extra-virgin olive oil

1. Preheat the broiler. Cover a baking sheet with aluminum foil (for easy clean up) and set aside.

2. Place the chicken in a gallon-size plastic zip-top bag (leave the bag unsealed). Pound the thick end of the chicken thin with the flat side of a meat mallet to create a chicken breast with uniform thickness.

3. Remove chicken from the bag and place it on the prepared baking sheet. Brush the chicken with oil on both sides. Sprinkle with seasoning mix and rub to evenly distribute.

4. Broil the chicken 6 inches from the heat source for 4 minutes on each side or until done (chicken is done when the internal temperature registers 165°F on a meat thermometer). Sprinkle the chicken with herbs immediately when removed from the oven. The heat will lightly cook the herbs.

Yield: 6 servings
(3 ounces)

Nutrient Breakdown:
Calories 150

Fat 5g (1g saturated fat, 3.5g monounsaturated fat)

Cholesterol 75mg

Sodium 130mg

Carbohydrate 0g

Fiber 0g

Protein 24g

Plate Plan choices:
3 very lean meats

*To freeze, wrap cooled chicken in freezer paper or place it in a plastic freezer bag; remove as much air as possible. Store the wrapped meat in another freezer bag (for extra protection). Be sure to write the contents and date on the outer bag. Cooked chicken will keep well in the freezer for up to 6 months.

pasta (or barley) salad florentine

Lunch Leftovers

Full of nutrition and flavor, this is a great addition to any potluck. While recipe testing, we tried this with 1 cup cooked barley instead of pasta: delicious. You will love this either way you try it. It also makes a great "Lunch Leftover" when you add previously prepared grilled chicken, fish or pork.

4 ounces whole-wheat farfalle (bow-tie) pasta (generous 3 cups, uncooked)

1 cup (½ pint) grape tomatoes, halved or quartered

1 cucumber, coarsely chopped

2 cups of roughly chopped fresh baby spinach (about 1½ ounces)

½ cup crumbled feta cheese (2 ounces)

1 teaspoon Jane's Krazy Mixed-Up Salt

2 tablespoons lemon juice

1 tablespoon extra-virgin olive oil

4 large basil leaves, chopped

GROCERY LIST:
Fresh basil leaves (4 leaves)

Cucumber (1)

Grape tomatoes (½ pint)

Fresh baby spinach (1½ ounces)

Lemon juice (2 tablespoons)

Whole-wheat farfalle pasta (half of an 8-ounce box)

Feta cheese

Jane's Krazy Mixed-Up Salt

Extra-virgin olive oil

Hands-on time: 20 minutes
Total time: 1 hour and 20 minutes (including refrigerator time)

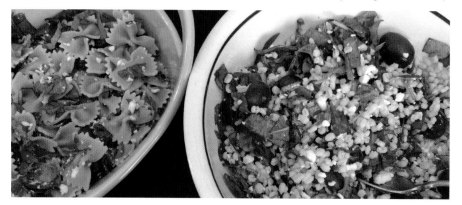

1. Cook pasta according to package directions until it is al dente (firm to bite).

2. While the pasta is cooking, place the tomatoes, cucumber, and spinach in a large bowl. Once the pasta is cooked, drain and rinse it briefly with cool water. Add warm pasta to the vegetables and mix to combine (the pasta should be a little warm to lightly cook the vegetables but not so warm that it melts the feta cheese in the next step).

3. Add the feta cheese, salt, juice, oil, and basil. Gently mix to combine. Refrigerate for 1–2 hours to let the flavors blend and allow the pasta to cool completely. Garnish with fresh basil leaves just before serving, if desired.

Yield: 6 servings
(serving size: ¾ cup)

Nutrient Breakdown:
Calories 130

Fat 4.5g (1.5g saturated fat)

Cholesterol 5mg

Sodium 300mg

Carbohydrates 17g

Fiber 3g

Protein 5g

Plate Plan choices:
1 vegetable, 1 starch, 1 fat

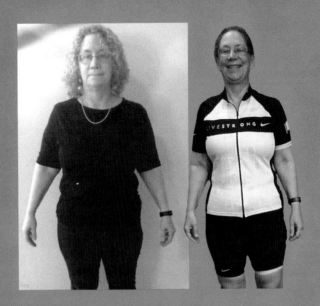

"I followed along each day and lost weight without feeling deprived. Over a few months, I lost 17 pounds and my husband lost 34 pounds eating what I prepare. We both learned a lot!

—KAREN, 54

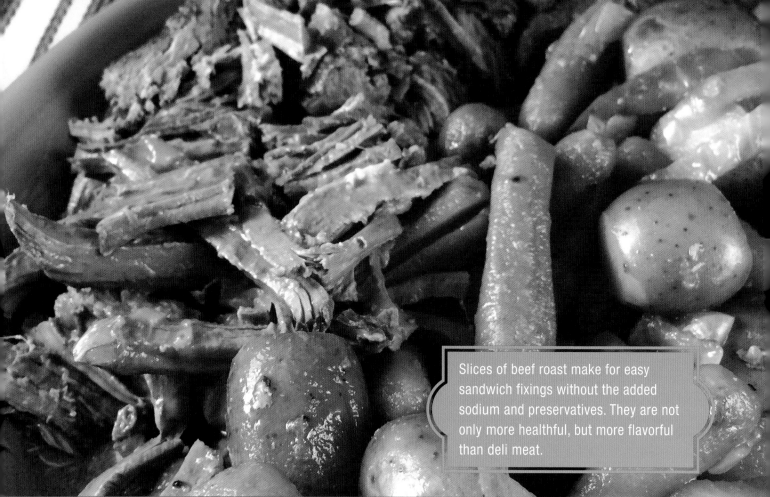

Slices of beef roast make for easy sandwich fixings without the added sodium and preservatives. They are not only more healthful, but more flavorful than deli meat.

DAY 19

Easy Meal

Slow-Cooker

easy slow-cooker beef roast dinner

Lunch Leftovers

A traditional roast that's perfect for Sunday dinner or a quick hearty weeknight meal. This also makes a great "Lunch Leftover."

suggested side: green salad

Hands-on time: 10 minutes
Total time: 8 hours and 10 minutes

1 10.5-ounce can golden mushroom soup

1 can water (refill empty soup can)

½ teaspoon fresh cracked black pepper

1 pound baby carrots

1 pound baby red potatoes left whole, or larger ones cut in half

1 large onion, sliced

1½ pounds top round roast, sirloin roast, or London broil, trimmed of excess fat

GROCERY LIST:
Onion (1 large)

Baby carrots (1 pound)

Baby red potatoes (20 or about 1 pound)

Top round roast, sirloin roast, or London broil (1½ pounds)

Golden mushroom soup (10.5-ounce can)

Black pepper

Salad fixings (suggested side)

1. Pour the soup and water into the slow cooker, then add the pepper and whisk together until creamy and no lumps remain.

2. Place the carrots and potatoes and half of the sliced onions over the bottom of the cooker, then place the meat* on top. Spoon liquid over the meat, making sure it is mostly covered with liquid (add a little more water if needed). Add the rest of the onions and cover.

3. Cook on low for about 8–10 hours or high for 5 hours (low and slow for optimal tenderness).

Yield: 6 servings
(serving size: about 3 ounces of beef and 1½ cups vegetables)

Nutrient Breakdown:
Calories 280

Fat 6g (2g saturated fat)

Cholesterol 70mg

Sodium 380mg

Carbohydrate 26g

Fiber 4g

Protein 26g

Plate Plan choices:
1 starch, 2 vegetables, 3 lean meats

*You can shred or cut the meat after it is done and return it to the cooker to soak in the juices while you make the salad.

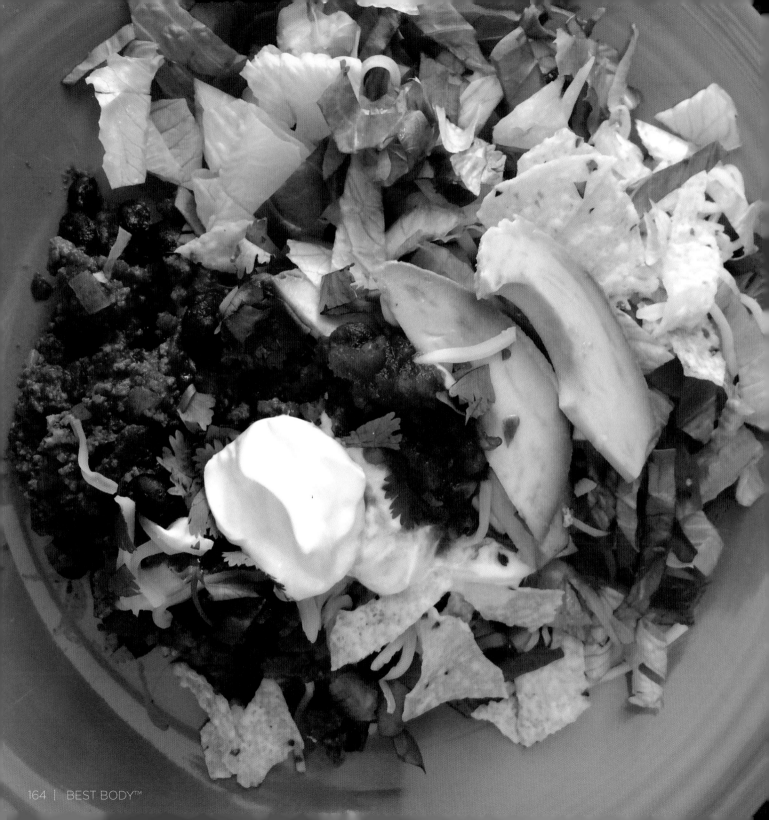

recipes & menu:
week six

> "Knowing is not enough, we must apply. Being willing is not enough, we must do!"
>
> —GOETHE

menu key:

Lunch Leftovers

Pricey Meal

Quicker-Fix

Slow-Cooker

Club Favorite

Easy Meal

DAY 18
Flounder with Tarragon Aioli
Sautéed Spinach and Tomatoes
Suggested side: barley

DAY 17
Chipotle Chicken Butternut Stew
Suggested side: green salad or raw veggies and hummus

DAY 16
Taco Salad

DAY 15
Chicken and Bok Choy Stir-fry
Suggested side: edamame

DAY 14
Zucchini Boats

DAY 13
Grilled Balsamic Pork Tenderloin
Carolina Salad
Roasted Brussels Sprouts and Carrots
Grilled Whole-Grain Bread

DAY 12
Spice-Rubbed Salmon on the Grill
Watermelon Feta Salad
Suggested side: grilled corn on the cob

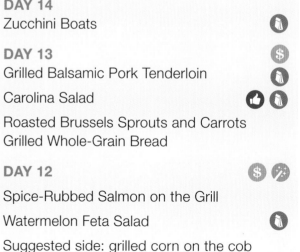

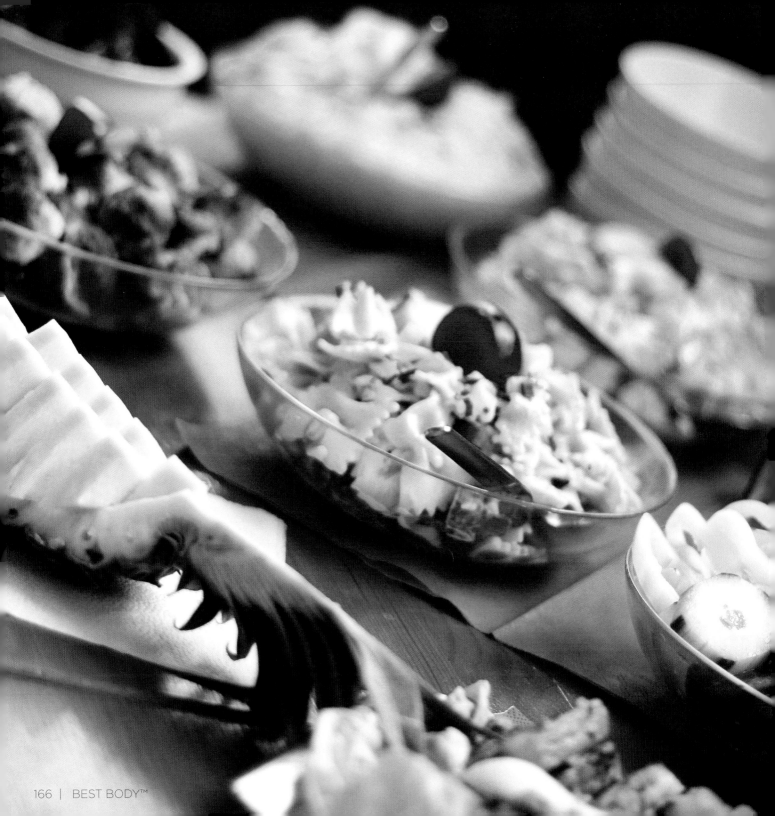

By the end of this week, you will have had the chance to utilize six weeks of recipes. We hope many of them have become new favorites in your home as you have been counting down to **Your Best Body**™, and we expect that there are still some you have not yet tried.

If you are like most people, you may eat the same 5–10 meals regularly, whether it's intentionally planned or not. Towards the end of this week, you will be asked to make a dinner menu plan to wrap up the last two weeks of the Countdown. This is to set you up with a strategy to help you maintain **Your Best Body**™ when the 52-day journey is complete. So, over the course of this week, you'll want to be brainstorming which recipes should become part of your regular meal rotation.

You will find a meal-planning template you can use in Appendix C, or you can type your plan in the interactive Menu Planner download (available at bestbodyin52.com/shop).

5 vegetable and fruit servings or more daily

4 cook-at-home meals weekly+

3 "Strategic Splurges" per week

2 meals from 1 (double recipes)

1 hour of pre-prep and planning time weekly

Easy Meal

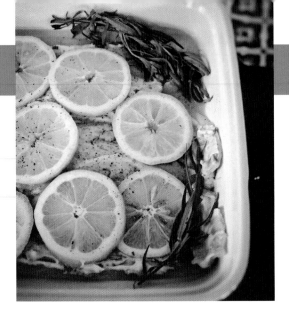

flounder with tarragon aioli

This is delicious, easy and elegant. You'll want to make it every week.

Canola oil cooking spray

4 4-ounce fresh or frozen flounder fillets (soak or thaw in milk, if desired)

¼ cup canola mayonnaise

2 teaspoons Dijon mustard

1 garlic clove, minced

2 teaspoons chopped fresh tarragon (or ½ teaspoon dried)

1 lemon, thinly sliced

Cracked black pepper, to taste

½ cup dry white wine (such as chardonnay)

1–2 additional tarragon sprigs (optional)

GROCERY LIST:

Fresh tarragon (fresh preferred, dried is a suitable substitute)

Garlic clove (1)

Lemon (1)

Flounder (4 4-ounce fresh or frozen fillets)

Canola mayonnaise

Dijon mustard

Dry white wine such as chardonnay (½ cup)

Cracked black pepper

Canola oil cooking spray

Barley (suggested side)

Hands-on time: 10 minutes
Total time: 25 minutes (allow frozen fish to thaw overnight in the refrigerator)

suggested side: barley

1. Preheat the oven to 375°F. Coat a 9x13-inch baking dish with cooking spray, and set aside.

2. Pat fish dry with paper towels. While gathering ingredients, allow the fish to rest on paper towels to soak up any remaining moisture (the more liquid soaked up in this step the better, as it will allow the sauce to soak in and flavor the fish during cooking).

3. To make aioli, combine the next 4 ingredients (mayonnaise through tarragon) in a small bowl and mix.

4. Place fish in the prepared baking dish. Top each fish fillet with a thin layer of aioli sauce and a lemon slice, reserving the remaining sauce and lemon to serve with the fish.

5. Sprinkle the fish with pepper. Gently pour the wine over the fish and add 1 sprig of tarragon to the liquid. Bake for 10–15 minutes or until done. Serve with reserved sauce and lemon.

Yield: 4 servings
(serving size: 1 fillet)

Nutrient Breakdown:
Calories 180

Fat 6g (0g saturated fat, 430mg omega-3 fatty acids)

Cholesterol 45mg

Sodium 350mg

Carbohydrate 3g

Protein 22g

Plate Plan choices:
3 very lean meats, ½ fat

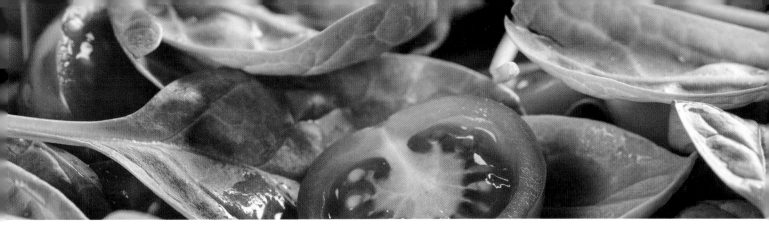

sautéed spinach and tomatoes

Total time: 10 minutes

Club Favorite

This simple recipe can be added to a bowl of grains with a lean protein for a quick meal anytime.

Canola oil cooking spray

1 tablespoon extra-virgin olive oil

4 cloves garlic, minced

1 pint grape tomatoes, halved

1 10-ounce package fresh baby spinach

$\frac{1}{8}$ teaspoon salt

Cracked black pepper to taste

GROCERY LIST:
Garlic cloves (4)

Grape tomatoes (1 pint)

Fresh baby spinach (10 ounces)

Black pepper

Salt

Extra-virgin olive oil

Canola oil cooking spray

1. Spray a large pot or Dutch oven with cooking spray and add oil. Place over medium heat. Once the oil is hot, add garlic and sauté for 30 seconds or until aromatic.

2. Add the tomatoes to the pan and sauté for 3 minutes. Add the spinach, salt and pepper. Using tongs or a pair of wooden spoons, toss the tomatoes and spinach together, making sure all get evenly coated with oil.

3. Cook, stirring occasionally for 2–3 minutes until the spinach is wilted.

Yield: 4 servings
(serving size: 1 cup)

Nutrient Breakdown:
Calories 50

Fat 2.5g (2g monounsaturated fat)

Cholesterol 0mg

Sodium 125mg

Carbohydrate 8g

Fiber 4g

Protein 2g

Plate Plan choices:
2 vegetables, ½ fat

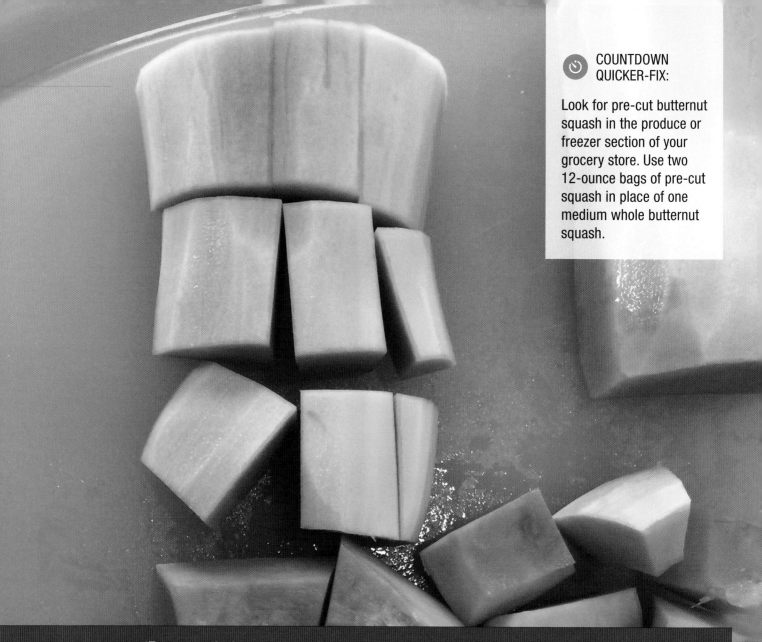

⏱ COUNTDOWN
QUICKER-FIX:

Look for pre-cut butternut squash in the produce or freezer section of your grocery store. Use two 12-ounce bags of pre-cut squash in place of one medium whole butternut squash.

*To prepare the butternut squash, begin by rinsing and drying the squash. Cut about ½-inch off of each end and then peel the skin off with a vegetable peeler. Next, carefully cut the neck away from the bulbous section. Place the squash so a cut end is on the cutting board and stable. Cut each section of the squash down the middle with a sharp, heavy knife (such as a chef's knife), then scrape the seeds out and discard. Lay the squash flat side down and cut into the desired size.

Slow-Cooker

chipotle chicken butternut stew

Quicker-Fix

Lunch Leftovers

This recipe is the perfect "Lunch Leftover." Try it over a bed of lettuce, as a taco salad, in tacos or just simply reheated. You'll love the warmth the chipotle chili contributes.

suggested side: green salad or raw veggies and hummus

Hands-on time: 30 minutes Total time: 8 hours and 20 minutes

1 medium onion, chopped (about 1½ cups)

1 medium butternut squash,* cut into ¾-inch pieces

1 red bell pepper, chopped (about 1 cup)

4 garlic cloves, minced

1½ pounds boneless, skinless chicken breasts

½ teaspoon salt

1 teaspoon dried oregano

2 tablespoons chili powder

½ teaspoon chipotle chili powder

½ teaspoon cumin

⅔ cup quinoa, rinsed

1 15-ounce can reduced-sodium black beans, drained and rinsed (or 1½ cups precooked beans)

1 14.5-ounce can no-salt-added petite diced tomatoes

2½ cups unsalted chicken broth

2 tablespoons chopped fresh cilantro (optional)

1. Place the onion, squash, red pepper, and garlic into the slow cooker.

2. Trim any remaining fat off of the chicken, lay it on top of the vegetables in the slow cooker, and sprinkle with seasonings (salt through cumin). Add the quinoa, black beans, tomatoes, and broth. Cook on high for 6 hours or on low for 8 hours. Serve with cilantro, if desired.

Yield: 6 servings
(serving size: 1½ cups)

Nutrient Breakdown:
Calories 340

Fat 4.5g (1g saturated fat)

Cholesterol 75mg

Sodium 490mg

Carbohydrate 45g

Fiber 9g

Protein 33g

Plate Plan choices:
2 starches, 2 vegetables, 4 very lean meats

GROCERY LIST:
Onion (1 medium)

Butternut squash (1 medium or 24 ounces pre-cut fresh or frozen)

Red bell pepper (1 cup chopped)

Garlic cloves (4)

Fresh cilantro (optional)

Boneless, skinless chicken breasts (1½ pounds)

Quinoa (⅔ cup)

Reduced-sodium black beans (1 15-ounce can)

No-salt-added petite diced tomatoes (1 14.5-ounce can)

Unsalted chicken broth

Salt

Oregano

Chili powder

Chipotle chili powder

Cumin

Salad fixings or raw veggies and hummus (suggested side options)

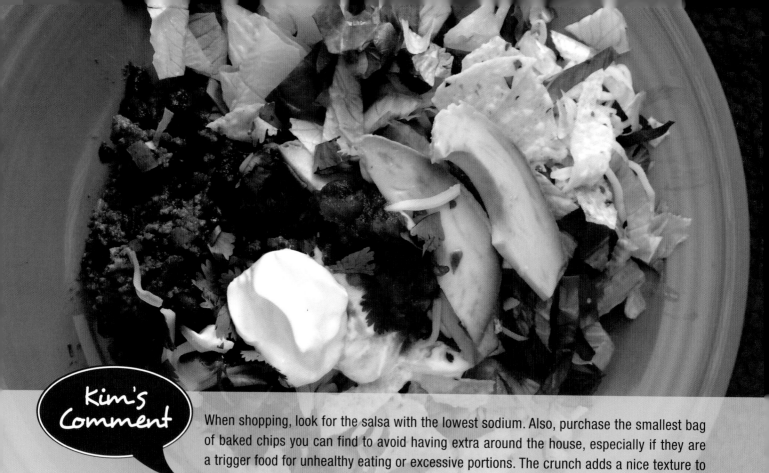

DAY 16

taco salad

This is a light, refreshing take on taco salad.

Total time: 30 minutes

MAKE THE MOST OF YOUR KITCHEN TIME: Double the meat and broth and use the entire taco seasoning packet. Freeze half for the next time you make this recipe or use for tacos another time.

1 teaspoon canola oil

½ cup finely chopped onion

2 garlic cloves, finely minced

1 pound lean ground beef (90% lean or leaner)

½ package reduced-sodium taco seasoning (just fold the top down twice to save for next time)

½ cup reduced-sodium broth (chicken, beef, or vegetable) or water

1 15-ounce can reduced-sodium pinto beans, drained and rinsed

½ cup roughly chopped fresh cilantro

2 large tomatoes, chopped (about 2 cups)

9 cups coarsely chopped romaine lettuce

1½ cups salsa (mild, medium or hot)

¾ cups shredded reduced-fat sharp cheddar cheese

6 tablespoons plain, nonfat Greek yogurt

6 tablespoons chopped green onions

1 avocado

¾ cup crumbled baked tortilla chips

1. Place a large nonstick skillet over medium heat and add oil. Once the oil is hot, add onions, garlic and ground beef. Break up the ground beef well with a wooden spoon or meat chopper. Once the meat begins to brown, add the taco seasoning packet and broth. Simmer for 8–10 minutes, stirring occasionally.

2. In a medium bowl, mix together the beans, cilantro, and tomatoes. Set aside.

3. To serve, place about 1½ cups of lettuce on each plate, top with ½ cup bean mixture, ½ cup meat, ¼ cup salsa, 2 tablespoons cheese, 1 tablespoon each of Greek yogurt and green onions, and a slice of avocado. Sprinkle with chips and enjoy.

Yield: 6 servings
(serving size: see step 3)

Nutrient Breakdown:
Calories 340

Fat 11g, (saturated Fat 4g)

Cholesterol 50mg

Sodium 640mg

Carbohydrate 28g

Fiber 7g

Protein 27g

Plate Plan choices:
1 starch,
2 vegetables, 2½ lean meats, 1 fat

GROCERY LIST:
Avocado (1)

Onion (1)

Garlic cloves (2)

Green onions

Fresh cilantro

Tomatoes (2 cups, chopped)

Romaine lettuce (9 cups, chopped)

Lean ground beef (1 pound)

Reduced-sodium broth

Reduced-sodium pinto beans

Salsa (1½ cups)

Reduced-fat sharp cheddar cheese

Plain, nonfat Greek yogurt

Reduced-sodium taco seasoning (1 package)

Canola oil

Baked tortilla chips

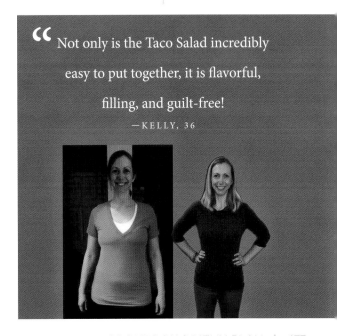

" Not only is the Taco Salad incredibly easy to put together, it is flavorful, filling, and guilt-free!

—KELLY, 36

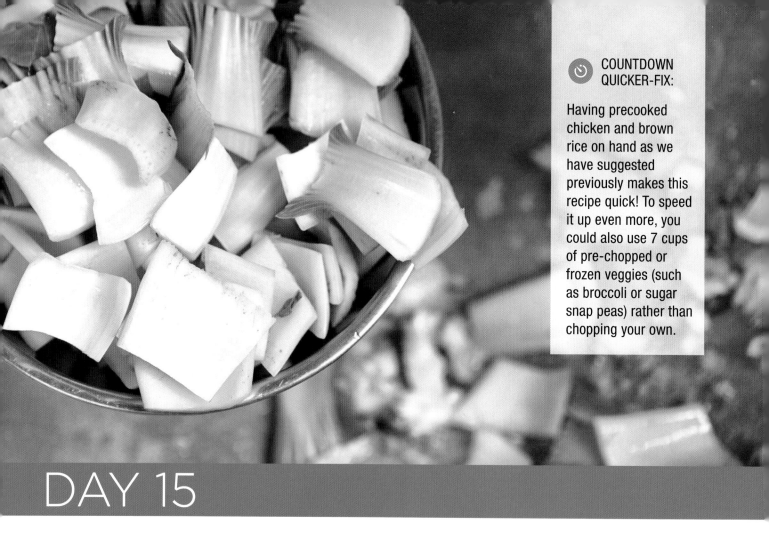

⏱ **COUNTDOWN QUICKER-FIX:**

Having precooked chicken and brown rice on hand as we have suggested previously makes this recipe quick! To speed it up even more, you could also use 7 cups of pre-chopped or frozen veggies (such as broccoli or sugar snap peas) rather than chopping your own.

DAY 15

chicken and bok choy stir-fry

Quicker-Fix   Lunch Leftovers

Bok choy is a unique and mild-tasting green. It cooks quickly and is a simple way to add more greens to your diet. Next time, try it with pork or shrimp for a twist. Either way, it is a recipe you will want to keep on hand.

The white stalks of the bok choy cook more slowly than the greens. Cooking them separately helps to keep the greens from over cooking.

suggested side:
edamame appetizer (1 cup)

Total time: 30 minutes

1 large head or 3–4 baby bok choy bunches (6 cups chopped bok choy)

Canola oil cooking spray

1 tablespoon canola oil

1 cup baby carrots, halved lengthwise (thick ones quartered)

1 small bunch green onions, chopped (green and white parts)

1½ tablespoons cornstarch

1 cup unsalted chicken or vegetable broth

2 tablespoons reduced-sodium soy sauce

1 teaspoon sesame oil

1 teaspoon grated ginger (or ginger from the tube)

1 clove garlic, minced

¾ pounds chopped precooked chicken (about 2¼ cups)

2 cups hot, cooked brown rice

1. Cut the ends off of the bok choy and separate. Rinse well (dirt can sometimes be trapped between leaves). Shake off excess water and stack the leaves. Cut the stems off and set aside. Next, cut the leaves in half along the stem line (while they are still stacked) and slice them across in 1-inch pieces. Keep the stems and leaves separated. Cut the stems into bite-sized pieces, discarding the bottom piece.

2. Coat a large nonstick skillet or pan with cooking spray, add oil, and place over medium-high heat. Once the oil is hot, swirl to coat the pan. Add carrots, bok choy stems and onions and stir-fry for 3 minutes.

3. Add the bok choy leaves to the pan and cook until the vegetables are crisp-tender, approximately 3 minutes.

4. As the greens cook, make the coating sauce. In a medium bowl, stir together the cornstarch and ¼ cup of chicken broth and mix until smooth. Add the remaining chicken broth, soy sauce, sesame oil, ginger and garlic and stir to combine.

5. Once the vegetables are cooked, add the chicken and coating sauce to the pan (if the sauce sits too long, it may be necessary to re-mix because the cornstarch will settle at the bottom).

6. Bring the mixture to a boil for a minimum of 1 minute and allow the sauce to thicken. Reduce the heat and cook until the chicken is heated through, about 3 minutes total. Serve over brown rice.

Yield: 4 servings
(serving size: 1½ cups chicken mixture and ½ cup rice)

Nutrient Breakdown:
(with 1 cup edamame):
Calories 310 (365)

Fat 8g (2g saturated, 4g monounsaturated fat)

Cholesterol 60mg

Sodium 590mg

Carbohydrate 35g (40g)

Fiber 5g (7g)

Protein 25g (30g)

Plate Plan choices:
2 starches,
2 vegetables,
3 very lean meats,
1 fat,
3 lean meats

GROCERY LIST:
Bok choy (1 large head or 3–4 baby bok choy bunches, 6 cups chopped)

Baby carrots (1 cup)

Green onions (1 bunch)

Garlic clove (1)

Ginger (1 teaspoon grated)

Precooked chicken (2¼ cups)

Brown rice, cooked (2 cups)

Unsalted chicken or vegetable broth

Cornstarch

Reduced-sodium soy sauce

Sesame oil

Canola oil

Canola oil cooking spray

Edamame, frozen in the pod (12 ounces, suggested side)

If using fresh chicken: cut the chicken into ¼-inch-wide bite-sized strips. Spray a large nonstick skillet with canola oil cooking spray, add ½ tablespoon canola oil, and place over medium-high heat. When the oil is hot, add the chicken to the pan and sauté for about 3 minutes or until done. With a slotted spoon or tongs, transfer the chicken to a plate; cover with aluminum foil to keep warm. Continue to prepare the recipe as directed.

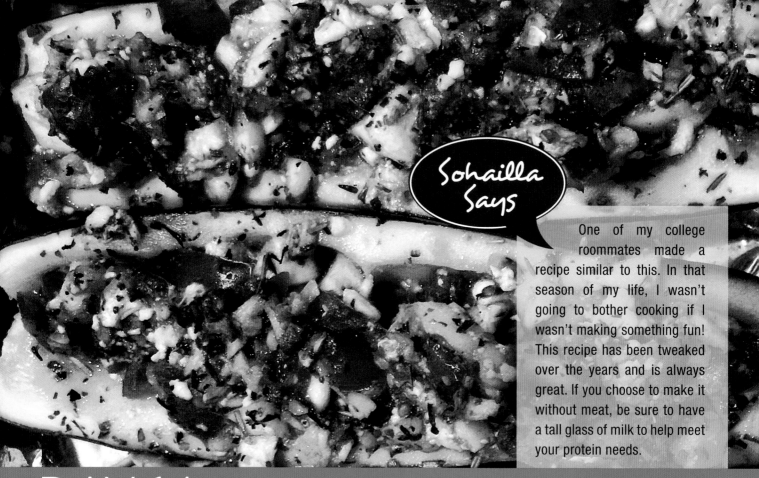

DAY 14

zucchini boats

Lunch Leftovers

This is a brilliant use of zucchini. It warms up nicely the next day, so if you plan to use it as a "Lunch Leftover," you may want to double the recipe.

Hands-on time: 20 minutes
Total time: 50 minutes

Cook black beans overnight on low in the slow cooker (6-8 hours) and store in 1-cup servings in ziptop bags in the freezer. Perfect for salads, soups, and this recipe!

2 large zucchinis

¾ cup reduced-fat shredded sharp cheddar cheese, divided

4 garlic cloves, minced

¾ cup chunky medium salsa

¼ teaspoon Jane's Krazy Mixed-Up Salt

1 cup black beans (use precooked or rinsed canned beans)

1 cup chopped cooked chicken (optional)

2 cups cooked quinoa, barley, or brown rice

GROCERY LIST:
Zucchini (2 large)

Garlic cloves (4)

Chicken (1 cup cooked, optional)

Quinoa, barley, or brown rice (2 cups cooked)

Chunky medium salsa

Black beans (1 cup, canned if not precooked)

Reduced-fat shredded sharp cheddar cheese

Jane's Krazy Mixed-Up Salt

1. Preheat the oven to 350°F. Cover a baking pan with aluminum foil (for easy clean-up) and set aside.

2. Wash and slice the zucchini lengthwise. Using a melon-ball scoop (or spoon), scoop the flesh out of the zucchini halves until they resemble a boat (carve close to the skin). Reserve the carved-out zucchini.

3. Chop the zucchini flesh and place in a medium bowl; mix with ¼ cup cheese, salsa, garlic, salt and beans (and chicken, if desired).

4. Spoon the mixture into the zucchini boats until very full. Top with the remaining ½ cup of cheese. Bake for 25–30 minutes. Serve over whole grains. For extra moisture and delicious flavor, drizzle the juices from the baking pan over the grain.

Yield: 4 servings
(serving size: 1 zucchini boat)

Nutrient Breakdown:
(with chicken):
Calories 250 (310)

Fat 7g (8g)

Cholesterol 15mg (45mg)

Sodium 610mg

Carbohydrate 38g

Fiber 7g

Protein 14g (25g)

Plate Plan choices:
1½ starches, 2 vegetables
1½ medium-fat meats
(chicken would add 1 lean meat)

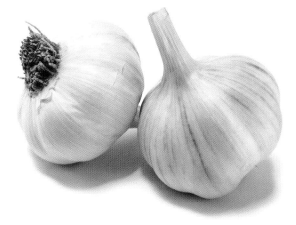

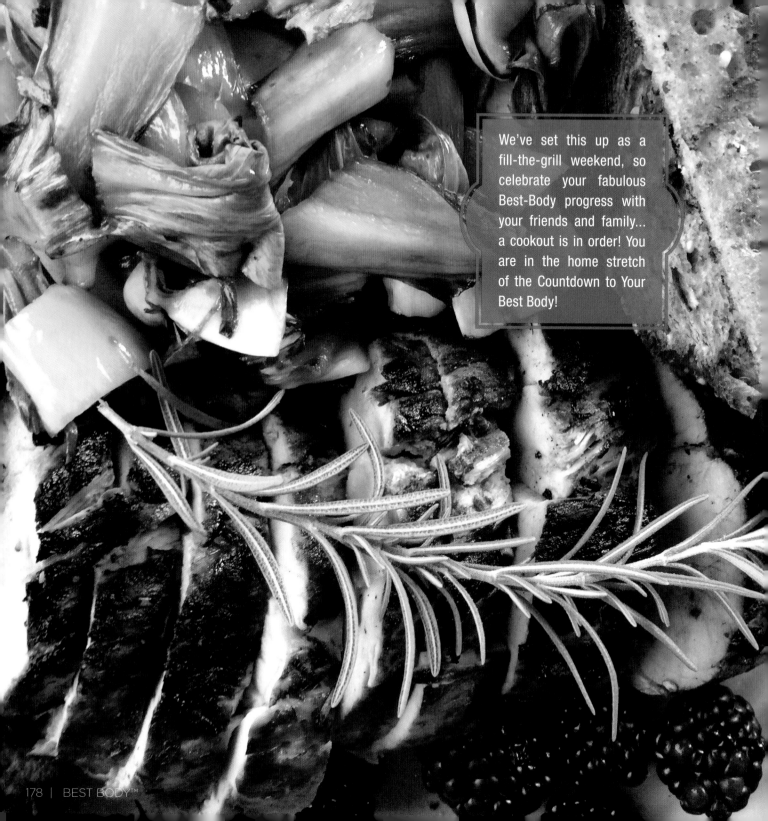

We've set this up as a fill-the-grill weekend, so celebrate your fabulous Best-Body progress with your friends and family... a cookout is in order! You are in the home stretch of the Countdown to Your Best Body!

Pricey Meal

grilled balsamic pork tenderloin

Lunch Leftovers

Club Favorite

This is simple and delicious. Pork tenderloin is about as lean as chicken breast, but it provides variety; it's a whole different taste and texture.

Hands-on time: 25 minutes   Total time: 1 hour and 25 minutes (includes 1 hour marinating time)

1 pound pork tenderloin

¼ cup balsamic vinegar

2 tablespoons extra-virgin olive oil

¼ teaspoon salt

¼ teaspoon cracked black pepper

1 teaspoon Dijon mustard

2 teaspoons honey

1 tablespoon fresh rosemary (or 1 teaspoon dried herbs of choice, such as oregano)

2 garlic cloves, minced or smashed into a paste (see procedure note on Day 28)

GROCERY LIST:
Pork tenderloin (1 pound)

Fresh rosemary (or fresh oregano or 1 teaspoon dried herbs of choice)

Garlic cloves (2)

Balsamic vinegar

Extra-virgin olive oil

Salt

Black pepper

Dijon mustard

Honey

1. Trim fat and silver skin (tough membrane with iridescent hue) from the pork tenderloin. To remove the silver skin, slip a knife blade between the silver skin and meat; angle the knife slightly upward, and use a gentle back-and-forth sawing motion to cut away the membrane.

2. Combine the vinegar and remaining ingredients in a gallon-sized plastic zip-top bag. Massage to mix the marinade. Add pork tenderloin, knead to cover pork with marinade, and marinate in the refrigerator for 1–3 hours.

3. When ready to cook, oil clean grill grates with a folded paper towel soaked in canola oil and preheat the grill to medium heat. Grill the tenderloin for 15 minutes, turning every 3–5 minutes until the internal temperature of the pork registers 145°F on a meat thermometer.

4. Remove from grill, tent with aluminum foil and let rest for 5–8 minutes before slicing (the meat will continue to cook with residual heat, and the juices will redistribute, making it more juicy).

Yield: 4 servings
(3 ounces)

Nutrient Breakdown:
Calories 160

Fat 6g (1.5g saturated fat, 4g monounsaturated fat)

Cholesterol 75mg

Sodium 250mg

Carbohydrate 2g

Added sugar 2g

Fiber 0g

Protein 24g

Plate Plan choices:
3 very lean meats, ½ fats

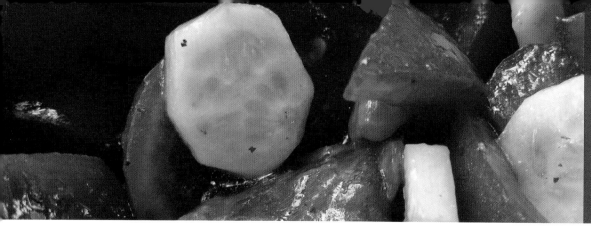

Go ahead and prepare a small portion of the vidalia onion and refrigerate for tomorrow: you'll need about 1 tablespoon, finely chopped or grated.

carolina salad

Hands-on time: 10 minutes
Total time: 40 minutes (including 30 minutes refrigerator time)

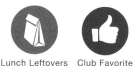

Lunch Leftovers   Club Favorite

Sohailla spent her twenties living on the Carolina coast; this is one of her favorite recipes from that time of life. It's simple and refreshing and always a crowd-pleaser!

3 medium tomatoes, cut into small chunks

2 large cucumbers or 5 pickling cucumbers, peeled and sliced, then halved

1 medium Vidalia onion, thinly sliced (about 1 cup)

½ cup white vinegar

1 tablespoon extra-virgin olive oil

¼ teaspoon salt

½ teaspoon black pepper

1. In a large salad bowl, gently stir tomatoes, cucumbers, and onions together, taking care to separate the onion pieces so that they resemble thin crescent moons.

2. In a small bowl, stir the remaining ingredients together (vinegar through pepper). Drizzle the dressing over the vegetables and stir gently. Place in the refrigerator while preparing the Grilled Whole-Grain Bread. Serve chilled.

Yield: 6 servings
(serving size: about 1 cup)

Nutrient Breakdown:
Calories 50

Fat 2.5g

Cholesterol 0mg

Sodium 105mg

Carbohydrate 6g

Fiber 2g

Protein 2g

Plate Plan choices:
2 vegetables

GROCERY LIST:

Tomatoes (3 medium)

Cucumbers (2 large) or pickling cucumbers (5)

Vidalia onion (1 medium)

White vinegar

Extra-virgin olive oil

Salt

Black pepper

roasted brussels sprouts and carrots

Brussels sprouts are under-appreciated and often overcooked. Both roasting and sautéing bring out the best in Brussels sprouts. Roasting them brings out a rich nutty flavor. The sauté method turns them bright green, highlighting their freshness, while the butter creates a luxurious mouthfeel.

Canola oil cooking spray

1 pound Brussels sprouts
(about 4 cups)

2 cups baby carrots (cut in half lengthwise or into quarters if they are thick)

1 medium onion, coarsely chopped (about 1 cup)

½ teaspoon dried thyme leaves
(or 1½ teaspoons fresh)

½ teaspoon Jane's Krazy Mixed-Up Salt

⅛ teaspoon black pepper

1 tablespoon extra-virgin olive oil

GROCERY LIST:

Brussels sprouts (1 pound or 4 cups)

Baby carrots (enough for 2 cups cut in half)

Onion (1 medium)

Dried thyme

Jane's Krazy Mixed-Up Salt

Black pepper

Extra-virgin olive oil (or butter for sauté method)

Canola oil cooking spray

Hands-on time: 10 minutes   Total time: 30 minutes

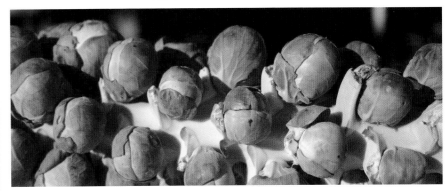

1. Preheat the oven to 400°F. Cover a baking pan in aluminum foil (for easy clean up) and spray with cooking spray.

2. Rinse Brussels sprouts, remove their outer leaves, and trim the stem end. Cut the small ones in half and the larger ones in quarters and place on the prepared baking pan. Add the carrots, onion, and seasonings to the pan and drizzle with oil. Toss the veggies to coat with seasonings and oil.

3. Spread the vegetables in a single layer and bake for 15–20 minutes or until done, turning once about halfway through cooking time to promote even browning.

Yield: 6 servings
(serving size: ¾ cup)

Nutrient Breakdown:
Calories 80

Fat 2.5g (1g saturated fat for the sautéed version)

Cholesterol 0mg

Sodium 140mg

Carbohydrates 12g

Fiber 4g

Protein 3g

Plate Plan choices:
2 vegetables

If you prefer to sauté, spray a large nonstick skillet with cooking spray and melt 1 tablespoon of butter over medium heat. Add the onion and carrot and sauté 4 minutes. Add Brussels sprouts and sauté 5 minutes or until crisp-tender. If the pan is a bit dry, add a couple tablespoons of water or chicken broth rather than more butter. Add thyme, salt and pepper and stir to mix thoroughly.

grilled whole-grain bread

Total time: 8 minutes

Although this resembles toast, it is better! Once you have the grill fired up, you may as well make the most of it. You'll love this alongside fresh tomatoes or any grilled vegetable.

2 cloves garlic, peeled and lightly smashed

4 thick slices whole-grain artisan bread (just over an ounce per slice)

2 tablespoons extra-virgin olive oil

¼ teaspoon salt (ideally coarse sea salt)

Chopped fresh herbs of choice (optional)

GROCERY LIST:
Fresh or dried herbs of choice (optional)

Garlic cloves (2)

Whole-grain artisan bread (4 thick slices)

Salt (ideally coarse sea salt)

Extra-virgin olive oil

1. Rub the garlic cloves lightly over the surface of the bread on both sides.
2. Brush both sides of the bread lightly with oil (you should only use about ½ the oil).
3. Grill the bread over medium-low heat for 1–1½ minutes per side, watching it carefully so it does not burn (a little char is great, too much is not).
4. Sprinkle with salt and fresh (or dried) herbs of choice, if desired.

Yield: 4 servings
(serving size: 1 slice)

Nutrient Breakdown:
Calories 110

Fat 5g

Cholesterol 0mg

Sodium 250mg

Carbohydrate 13g

Fiber 3g

Protein 3g

Plate Plan choices:
1 starch, 1 fat

Throw 2 more pieces of bread on the grill for making homemade croutons to go in tomorrow's Watermelon Feta Salad.

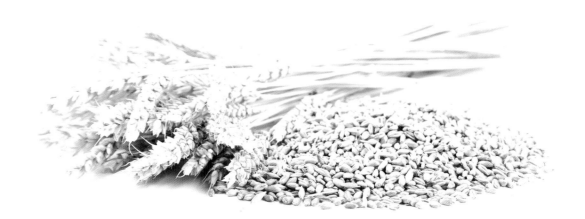

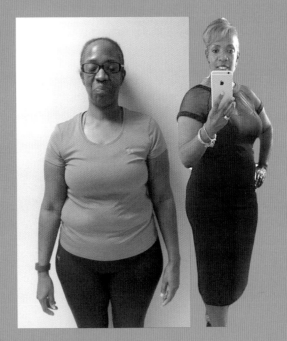

"The Best Body Countdown taught me the importance of planning meals -- the menus make it easy and the recipes are delicious. I feel great! I look forward to continuing my Best Body journey."

— CLAUDETTE, 53

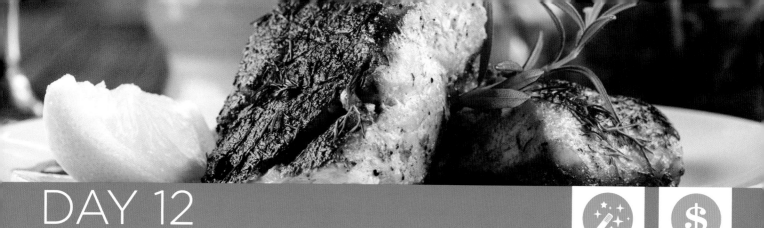

DAY 12

Easy Meal   Pricey Meal

spice-rubbed salmon on the grill

Total time: 15 minutes

If you have never been a big fan of salmon prepared traditionally (with garlic and lemon), you will enjoy the distinctively unique flavor of this recipe.
And for the salmon-lovers, this will be a new favorite!

suggested side: corn on the cob
(prepare on the grill alongside the salmon, carefully removing husks after the salmon is done)

1 lemon (juice plus 2 teaspoons grated lemon rind)

4 4-ounce salmon fillets, Pacific wild-caught preferred (soak or thaw in milk, if desired)

1 tablespoon brown sugar

3 teaspoons chili powder

¾ teaspoon cumin

½ teaspoon salt

¼ teaspoon cinnamon

GROCERY LIST:
1 lemon (zest and juice needed)

Salmon fillets (1 pound, Pacific wild-caught preferred)

Brown sugar

Chili powder

Cumin

Cinnamon

Salt

1. Zest the lemon and set the zest aside until you are ready to make the rub. Next, squeeze the juice of the lemon over the salmon and allow it to rest while you prepare tonight's dinner ingredients.

2. Oil clean grill grates with a folded paper towel soaked in canola oil and preheat the grill to medium-high heat.

3. In a small bowl, mix the seasonings to make the rub (brown sugar through cinnamon). Gently rub the seasoning mix onto the flesh side of the salmon, coating the top and sides.

4. Grill salmon fillets skin side down for 10 minutes or until cooked completely (the flesh will be opaque but will still be moist). Because this recipe uses a spice rub, we do not recommend flipping the salmon on the grill.

Yield: 4 servings
(serving size: 1 fillet)

Nutrient Breakdown:
Calories 180

Fat 7g (1g saturated fat, 6g monounsaturated fat, 1200mg omega-3 fatty acids)

Cholesterol 60mg

Sodium 370mg

Carbohydrate 5g

Protein 23g

Added Sugar 3g

Plate Plan choices:
3 lean meats

watermelon feta salad

Total time: 10 minutes

Lunch Leftovers

The saltiness of the feta cheese goes beautifully with the watermelon! This is delicious the next day, too, after the flavors meld together fully. That's why we set it up to make 8 servings (feel free to reduce the recipe by half).

---

1 tablespoon red wine vinegar

1 tablespoon grated Vidalia onion (or finely chopped)

1 teaspoon extra-virgin olive oil

7 cups cubed watermelon

1½ cups cubed English cucumber

1 cup crumbled feta cheese (4 ounces)

Cracked black pepper to taste

1 8-ounce bag romaine and radicchio salad mix (or other salad greens)

1½ cups homemade croutons (cubes cut from 2 slices of Grilled Bread, see Day 13)

1. If you have a large metal bowl, set it in the refrigerator to chill.

2. In a small bowl, combine vinegar, onion, and oil.

3. Place watermelon, cucumber and feta cheese in a chilled metal bowl and gently mix.

4. Drizzle with the dressing and toss with cracked pepper. (If you plan to enjoy this as a "Lunch Leftover" tomorrow, reserve some to refrigerate before adding it to the lettuce).

5. Serve watermelon mixture over the romaine and radicchio; top with croutons.

GROCERY LIST:

1 8-ounce bag romaine and radicchio salad mix (or other salad greens)

Vidalia onion (small)

Watermelon (1 medium for 7 cups cubed)

English cucumber (1)

Crumbled feta cheese (4 ounces)

Red wine vinegar

Cracked black pepper

Extra-virgin olive oil

Croutons (or use homemade)

Yield: 8 servings
(serving size: 1¾ cups)

Nutrient Breakdown:
Calories 80

Fat 3g (1.5g saturated fat)

Cholesterol 5mg

Sodium 180mg

Carbohydrate 11g

Fiber 1g

Protein 4g

Plate Plan choices:
1 veg, 1 fruit, 1 fat

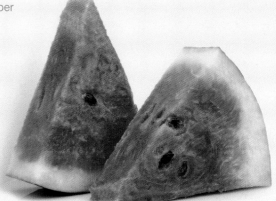

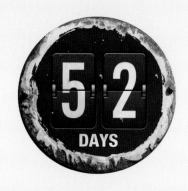

Have you tried some of the recipes but would say that you are not currently at Your Best Body? When you are ready to see and feel what your body is like at its best, we urge you to combine these flavor-packed recipes with the Best Body Countdown's principles, daily accountability, online support and success-tools for a fad-free tried and true pathway to Your Best Body.

We can't wait to hear from you! Share on the Best Body in 52 Facebook page.

Summary

We trust that you have discovered many new favorite recipes, and have learned lifelong Best-Body strategies along the way. Most people are surprised to find out how delicious and simple healthy recipes can be!

If you are participating in the Best Body Countdown, these last days of the 52 are critical to setting up your "healthfully ever after." Historically, the program participants who take the time to create their two-week menu plans are typically the "Best Body Superstars." They maintain their transformations, like those you have seen throughout the pages of this book, having adopted the five essentials we've practiced over the past six weeks.

Can you recall from memory the five essentials covered during this Cookbook Countdown? If so, perhaps it has become natural for you to visually divide your plate in half with the goal of prioritizing produce (remember the "happy half-a-plate?"). Maybe you now find yourself eating home-based meals more often -- saving your strategic splurges for when you feel they matter most. Have you been more mindful of which recipes work best for you to double? Have you set time aside consistently (typically about an hour) to prepare and plan for the week's menu? Keeping these five essentials in mind, along with the Countdown 5-4-3-2-1 essentials from the **Countdown to Your Best Body Success Journal**, sets the foundation for you to reach and maintain Your Best Body, without turning back to old habits.

References

Bissex, Janice Newell, and Liz Weiss. "Tips for Editing Beautiful Food Photos on Your Smart Phone (Part 2)." Meal Makeover Moms Kitchen. N.p., 24 Oct. 2014. Web. 24 May 2015. <http://mealmakeovermoms.com/kitchen/2014/10/24/edit-smart-phone-food-photos-with-snapseed/>.

"Is Canola Oil Healthy? - Nutrition Action." Nutrition Action. Nutrition Action, n.d. Web. 24 Nov. 2015. <http://www.nutritionaction.com/daily/fat-in-food/fat-in-food-the-truth-about-canola-oil/>.

"Cook with Canola or Olive Oil - Nutrition Action." Nutrition Action. Nutrition Action, n.d. Web. 24 Nov. 2015. <http://www.nutritionaction.com/daily/fat-in-food/cook-with-canola-or-olive-oil/>.

"Safe Minimum Internal Temperature Chart." USDA Food Safety and Inspection Service. USDA, n.d. Web. 24 Nov. 2015. <http://www.fsis.usda.gov/>.

Showell, Bethany A., Juhi R. Williams, MaryBeth Duvall, Juliette C. Howe, Kristine Y. Patterson, Janet M. Roseland, and Joanne M. Holden. "USDA Table of Cooking Yields for Meat and Poultry." www.ars.usda.gov. USDA, Dec. 2012. Web. June 2015. <http://www.ars.usda.gov/>.

Tribole, Evelyn. "Get Enough Long-Chain Omega-3 Fats in Your Diet." The Ultimate Omega-3 Diet: Maximize the Power of Omega-3s to Supercharge Your Health, Battle Inflammation, and Keep Your Mind Sharp. New York: McGraw-Hill, 2007. 139-58. Print.

Coconut oil:
Nutrition Action. Nutrition Action, n.d. Web. <http://www.nutritionaction.com/daily/fat-in-food/fat-in-food-the-truth-about-coconut-oil/>.

Cunningham, Eleese, RDN. "Is There Science to Support Claims for Coconut Oil." Eatrightpro. Academy of Nutrition and Dietetics, n.d. Web. 20 Nov. 2015. <http://www.eatrightpro.org/resource/news-center/nutrition-trends/foods-and-supplements/is-there-science-to-support-claims-for-coconut-oil>.

Chia Seed:
Bobs Red Mill. N.p., n.d. Web. 24 Nov. 2015. <http://www.bobsredmill.com/chia-seed.html>.

Food Equivalents:
"A to Z Food and Cooking Equivalents and Yields." About.com Food. N.p., n.d. Web. 24 Nov. 2015. <http://southernfood.about.com/library/info/blequivc.htm>.

Recipe writing:
Ostmann, Barbara Gibbs., and Jane L. Baker. The Recipe Writer's Handbook. New York: Wiley, 2001. Print.

Beavers, K.G. Eating Well with Kim. Retrieved from www.universityhealth.org/ewwk

Recipe Inspiration:
Toby Amidor, MS, RD nutrition expert and author of The Greek Yogurt Kitchen: More Than 130 Delicious, Healthy Recipes for Every Meal of the Day. www.tobyamidornutrition.com

Selected Resources:

Countdown to Your Best Body Success Journal." Charleston, South Carolina: Create Space, 2014. Print.

Academy of Nutrition and Dietetics

American Diabetes Association

American Heart Association

Center for Science in the Public Interest

Nutrition Action Healthletter

Index

Appendix A

Serving Sizes   hint: 1 grain or starch = 15 g carb; limit or avoid those along the bottom

Meats	Vegetables	Grain/Starch	Fruit	Dairy	Fat

Fish (not fried)
  Salmon, trout, herring, flounder, mackerel, tuna, and others
 	
Poultry:
  White meat, no skin
 	
Beef and Pork:
  Loin and round cuts are typically lean
 	
lean lunch meat (limit nitrates)
1 egg = 1 oz. meat
	1 cup raw vegetables
	½ cup cooked or finely chopped vegetables
	
	starchy vegetables and beans are counted with grains because of their starchy quality
		1/3 cup cooked rice
		
		1/2 cup cooked pasta , oats, quinoa, bulgur, or barley
		
		½ cup grits
		
		6 saltine-size crackers or 2 crisp-breads
		
		1 slice whole-grain bread (1 ounce)
		
		½ whole wheat pita or English muffin
		
		¾ cup whole-grain cereal
		
		1/2 cup of corn, peas, potatoes, sweet potatoes, or beans
			1 tennis ball–sized fruit such as an apple, peach, etc.
			
			½ banana
			
			¾ cup any berries
			
			1 cup any melon cubes
			
			½ cup applesauce, unsweetened
			
			2 tbsp. dried fruits
			
			4 ounces 100% juice
				1 cup skim or 1% milk
				
				1 cup yogurt, regular or Greek yogurt
				
				1.5 oz fat-free or reduced-fat cheese
				  Mozzarella, ricotta, and feta are naturally lower in fat
				
				¼ cup low-fat cottage cheese
					2 tbsp. avocado (1/5)
					8 olives
					4–10 nuts
					1 ½ tsp nut butter
					1 tbsp. sunflower, pumpkin, or flax seeds
					
					1 tsp. oil
					1 tbsp. Promise or Smart Balance spread
					1 tbsp. salad dress-ing (2 if tbsp. light) dressing
					
					2 tsp. mayo
					1 tsp. coconut oil
					1 tsp. butter
					1 tbsp. cream cheese

Avoid: Bologna, bacon, sausage, salami, hot dogs, and limit highly processed deli meats		Limit: White or refined grain products, biscuits, cornbread, granola, fried potatoes, waffles, cookies, and cakes	Limit: Juice, fruit drinks	Limit: Whole milk, full-fat cheeses and yogurts, ice cream, cream soups	Limit or Avoid: Butter, cream soups, stick margarine, bacon, fatback, gravy, cream, shortening, full-fat dressings, and hydrogenated oils (trans fat) in packaged products

Appendix B

My BEST BODY Shopping List (think perimeter!)

Fresh produce (did you get all colors of the rainbow?)

_____   _____
_____   _____
_____   _____
_____   _____
_____   _____

Lean protein (fish, poultry & round/loin cuts of pork/beef or tofu)

_____   _____
_____   _____
_____   _____
_____   _____
_____   _____

Whole grains, cereals and beans

_____   _____
_____   _____
_____   _____
_____   _____

Low sodium canned goods and dried fruits

_____   _____
_____   _____

Dairy, eggs, and frozen foods

_____   _____
_____   _____
_____   _____
_____

Appendix C

MEAL PLANNING	PICTURE IT!	GROCERY NEEDS	PREPARATION TIPS
Monday's Dinner			
Tuesday's Dinner			
Wednesday's Dinner			
Thursday's Dinner			
Friday's Dinner			
Saturday's Dinner			
Sunday's Dinner			

Appendix D

FOOD LOG DATE: _____	WHEN AND WHERE?	HUNGER BEFORE AND SATIETY AFTER
BREAKFAST		0 1 2 3 4 5 6 7 8 9 10 Starving Content Stuffed 0 1 2 3 4 5 6 7 8 9 10 Starving Content Stuffed
SNACK		0 1 2 3 4 5 6 7 8 9 10 Starving Content Stuffed
LUNCH		0 1 2 3 4 5 6 7 8 9 10 Starving Content Stuffed 0 1 2 3 4 5 6 7 8 9 10 Starving Content Stuffed
SNACK		0 1 2 3 4 5 6 7 8 9 10 Starving Content Stuffed
DINNER		0 1 2 3 4 5 6 7 8 9 10 Starving Content Stuffed 0 1 2 3 4 5 6 7 8 9 10 Starving Content Stuffed
NOTES:		

☐ I REACHED MY WATER GOAL!

Appendix E

Shopping Staples

FRESH PRODUCE (ALL!)

- ☑ Salad greens
- ☑ Bagged rainbow slaw (also called California slaw or broccoli slaw)
- ☑ Garlic (fresh, in the tube or minced)
- ☑ Onions (onions are storage produce and last a long time in the crisper drawer)
- ☑ Carrots (carrots last a long time in the refrigerator)
- ☑ Apples (Apples keep well in the crisper drawer)
- ☑ Seasonal farmer's market specials

LEAN MEATS

- ☑ Fish
- ☑ Chicken and turkey breast
- ☑ Lean pork and beef (loin or round cuts)
- ☑ Canned tuna and salmon

WHOLE GRAINS, CEREALS, AND BEANS

- ☑ Canned reduced-sodium beans and bagged dry beans (black, pinto, navy, kidney, etc.)
- ☑ Whole grains (brown rice, whole-wheat pasta, barley, quinoa, old-fashioned or steel cut oats, etc.)
- ☑ Whole-grain pitas
- ☑ Ezekiel cinnamon-raisin English muffins

LOW-SODIUM CANNED GOODS AND DRIED FRUITS

- ☑ No-salt-added canned tomatoes (diced, stewed, and with green chilis)
- ☑ Reduced-sodium and unsalted stock or broth (chicken, vegetable, beef)
- ☑ Raisins (golden and purple)

DAIRY, EGGS, AND FROZEN FOODS

- ☑ Milk (1% or nonfat), plain soymilk or almond milk
- ☑ Eggs
- ☑ Butter or trans-fat-free spread
- ☑ Greek yogurt (plain, nonfat)
- ☑ Frozen fruit (blueberries, strawberries, blackberries, peaches)
- ☑ Frozen vegetables (stir-fry blends, mirepoix, chopped onions and peppers)
- ☑ Frozen chicken or fish (non-breaded)

MISCELLANEOUS

- ☑ Spice blends (Mrs. Dash salt-free seasonings, Jane's Krazy Mixed-Up Salt, Cavendar's Greek seasoning, grill seasonings, Italian seasoning, etc.)
- ☑ Healthy oil (canola oil, extra-virgin olive oil, canola oil cooking spray)
- ☑ Dressings such as Newman's Own Balsamic Vinegar and Bolthouse Farms Greek Yogurt Dressing
- ☑ Nuts and nut butter such as peanut butter or almond butter

Appendix F

FOOD	SERVING SIZE	FIBER (GRAMS)
pear with skin*	1 medium	5.5 grams
apple with skin*	1 medium	4.4 grams
strawberries*	3/4 cup	3.0 grams
orange*	1 medium	3.1 grams
whole wheat pasta	1/2 cup	3.2 grams
barley, cooked*	1/2 cup	3.0 grams
bran flakes*	3/4 cup	5.3 grams
oatmeal*, cooked	1 cup	4.0 grams
popcorn, air-popped	3 cups	3.5 grams
lentils*	1/2 cup	8 grams
lima beans*	1/2 cup	7 grams
baked beans*	1/3 cup	3.5 grams
green peas*	1/2 cup	4.4 grams
navy beans*	1/2 cup	6 grams
kidney beans*	1/2 cup	6 grams
broccoli	1/2 cup	2.6 grams
brussels sprouts*	1/2 cup	3.0 grams

*denotes soluble fiber-rich foods

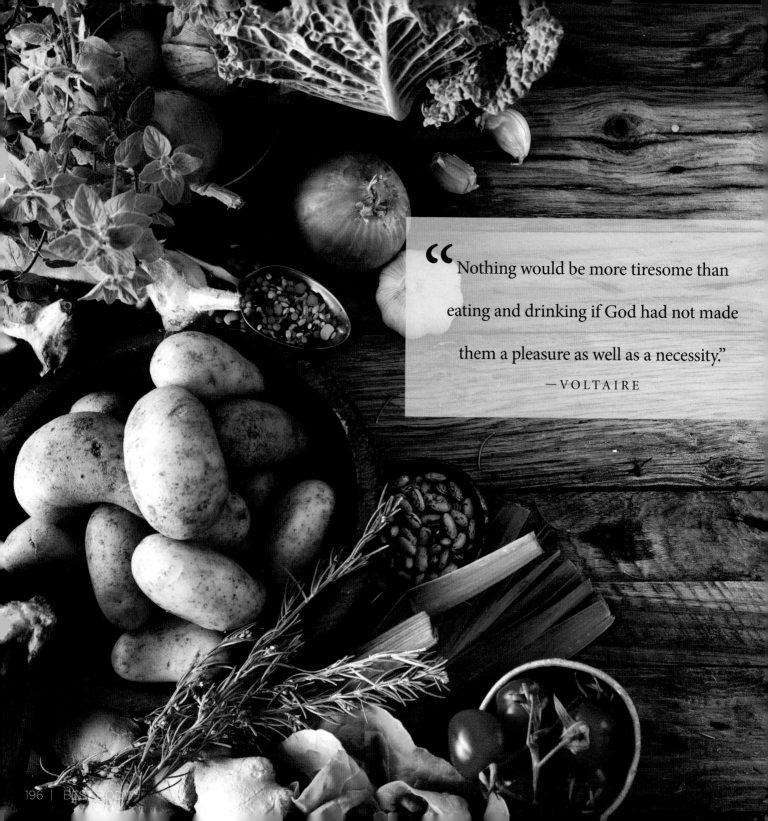

"Nothing would be more tiresome than eating and drinking if God had not made them a pleasure as well as a necessity."

—VOLTAIRE

Acknowledgments

We were acquaintances at best when we started to write this book together, but each met our match in grit; both of us equally willing to persevere through more details than we ever imagined... and harmoniously, too! We are grateful to each other for committed teamwork and friendship, and we acknowledge God graciously allowed our paths to cross at this juncture and is the giver of anything noteworthy that we have to offer.

Our designer has been a gem -- doing the finishing work to create a book that is as beautiful as it is all-inclusive. One that beckons you to choose healthy food while supporting you in staying the Best-Body course. Thank you Summer, for your tireless work to make our words look as lovely as the recipes taste.

We are deeply grateful for our precious husbands who support us and share life's loads with us. Without them we could not accomplish pieces of work such as this in order to enrich and extend lives, and strengthen bodies and families. Many thanks to our children for tasting recipes, helping clean up Mommy's messes in the kitchen, and for timely hugs on the long editing days.

We appreciate our dear friends, family members, and fans: testing recipes, proofing documents, lending a hand, and cheering us on while excitedly awaiting the finish line of this project. Our dietitian colleagues and the Best Body Nutrition & Fitness team have been a wealth of support in this endeavor as well. We are blessed!

Last but not least, we applaud the thousands of clients and readers that have had the determination to finish out the Best Body Countdown's 52-day journey (and the boldness to insist on a menu plan to complement it). Thank you for allowing us to share tidbits from your personal experiences and your recipe favorites. Your progress is inspiring...our hope is that these recipes and tips become part of your Best-Body success story.

About the Authors
SOHAILLA DIGSBY

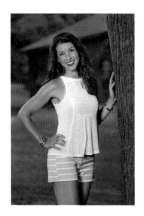

Sohailla Digsby is a registered dietitian nutritionist, fitness instructor, national speaker and author of the **Countdown to Your Best Body Success Journal**. She is the Founder of Best Body Nutrition & Fitness, LLC, supporting facilitators around the nation in using her 52-day Best Body Countdown™ program to affect lifestyle change.

Sohailla has been teaching fitness since beginning her nutrition studies about 20 years ago. Over her years of experience as a dietitian and fitness pro, she has learned that just as exercise regimens must be enjoyable to be adhered to regularly, meals must be flavorful and balanced for people to make lasting changes in their eating habits.

On a typical day you might find her in heels giving a presentation, later in sneakers jogging alongside her kids as they bike in the neighborhood while a slow-cooker dinner simmers, and then around the table with her family in her slippers. Sohailla prioritizes making health, food, and fitness both fun and practical so that you will be compelled to do the same for the long-haul!

Sohailla is an award-winning dietitian, holding a Dietetics degree from the University of Georgia, with honors. She completed her post-graduate dietetic internship in Augusta, Georgia, close to where she currently resides with her husband of 17 years and 3 children. As a member of the Academy of Nutrition and Dietetics (AND), she actively participates in the Nutrition Entrepreneurs and Weight Management AND practice groups, and is also an ACE-certified fitness instructor. She is passionate about keeping her message balanced and realistic, knowing that after the hype of the fads fade, people need practical steps, wholesome, delicious recipes, and accountability to stay the Best-Body course.

Check out Sohailla's Countdown to Your Best Body Success Journal *to pair with this Cookbook & Menu Plan to reach Your Best Body in 52 days! And be sure to watch for the next accompanying publication to the Success Journal and Cookbook to learn more about why Sohailla chose exactly 52 days for the Countdown. Stay in touch through bestbodyin52.com.*

About the Authors
KIM BEAVERS

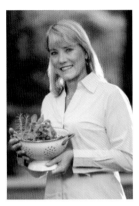

Kim has been writing and talking about food throughout her 20-year career as a registered dietitian nutritionist. For the past ten years she has been the producer and co-host of University Health Care System's culinary nutrition segment *Eating Well with Kim*, which airs three times a week on local television. Several of the recipes included in this book originated as *Eating Well with Kim* recipes. In addition, Kim writes a regular column for the Augusta Family Magazine, highlighting favorite recipes and nutrition topics.

Demonstrating recipes on air has allowed her to hone her recipe development and presentation skills. One of Kim's passions is to show viewers that eating healthfully is delicious. As a "picky eater" in her youth, Kim developed a natural appreciation for the importance of flavor. She believes strongly that healthy food must taste good in order for eating habits to change. Just as form follows function, so too does nutrition follow flavor. You can be sure that Kim did not eat "yucky" food as a child, does not eat it now, nor will she suggest that you do. Pass the flavor please!

Kim is an award-winning dietitian and holds a Bachelor and Master of Science degree in Health Sciences from James Madison University. She is a Certified Diabetes Educator and a member of the Academy of Nutrition and Dietetics (AND). She actively participates in several AND practice groups including the Food and Culinary Professionals, Diabetes Care and Education, and Nutrition Entrepreneurs groups. She enjoys sharing her nutrition expertise with others and is delighted with the growing interest in fresh local food. After all, fresh food is more flavorful.

Kim enjoys an active lifestyle which includes tennis, running, biking and various fun adventures with her husband of 14 years, 2 energetic children, and family dog.

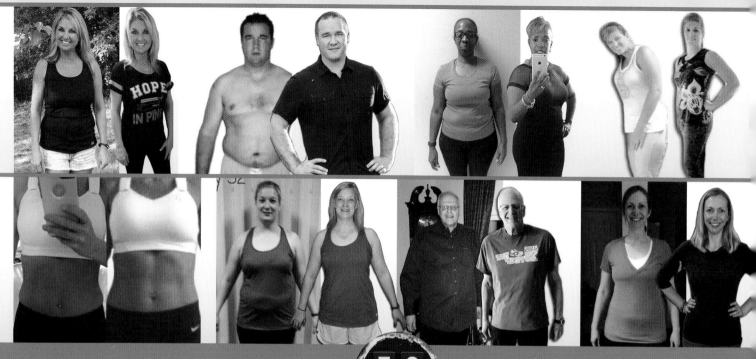

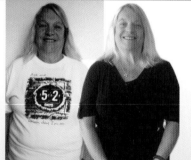
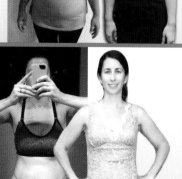
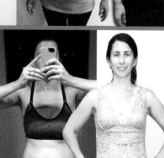
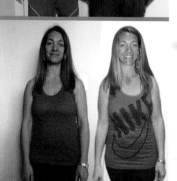
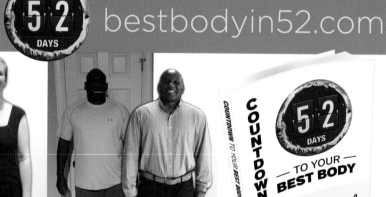

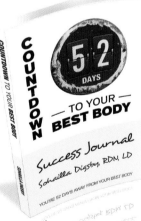